Independent and Supplementary Prescribing

An Essential Guide

To

Tim, Tom and Kath. The last book . . . . . . maybe
Donna, Hope and Oscar. The last book . . . . . . definitely

Independent and Supplementary Prescribing
An Essential Guide

Edited by

Molly Courtenay
*Reader, Prescribing & Medicines Management, School of Health &
Social Care, University of Reading
Joint Prescribing Adviser, RCN*

Matt Griffiths
*Senior Lecturer, Prescribing, School of Health Studies,
Homerton College, Cambridge
Joint Prescribing Adviser, RCN*

Foreword by

Dr June Crown CBE
*Chairman, Review of the Prescribing, Supply and
Administration of Medicines*

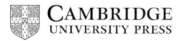

CAMBRIDGE
UNIVERSITY PRESS

CAMBRIDGE UNIVERSITY PRESS

Cambridge, New York, Melbourne, Madrid, Cape Town, Singapore, São Paulo

CAMBRIDGE UNIVERSITY PRESS
The Edinburgh Building, Cambridge CB2 2RU, UK

Published in the United States of America by Cambridge University Press, New York

www.cambridge.org
Information on this title: www.cambridge.org/9780521674645

First published 2004
Reprinted 2005

Printed in the United Kingdom at the University Press, Cambridge

A catalogue record for this book is available from the British Library

ISBN-13 978-0-521-67464-6 paperback
ISBN-10 0-521-67464-6 paperback

Contents

Foreword

The extension of the authority to prescribe has moved on apace since the publication of the Review of the Prescribing, Supply and Administration of Medicines in 1999. Now nurses and pharmacists, as well as doctors and dentists, can prescribe, and they will soon be joined by other health professionals. These rapid developments have set challenges for professional and regulatory bodies and for individual practitioners. However, all concerned have risen to these challenges with energy and enthusiasm. Training programmes are well developed, many nurses and pharmacists have completed training, and the benefits to patients are already being felt.

This book is timely and I would like to congratulate Molly Courtenay and Matt Griffiths on bringing together a group of distinguished contributors who have produced an authoritative and comprehensive account of all aspects of prescribing. I am sure that it will prove invaluable both as a practical guide to new prescribers and a continuing reference source.

I hope that this book will not be seen only as a book for the new prescribing professions. Its thorough examination of all aspects of the prescribing process and the implications of extended prescribing for multidisciplinary teams should also commend it to existing prescribers. It is a valuable text for every professional who is learning to prescribe or who wishes to improve their practice.

I have no doubt that *Independent* and *Supplementary Prescribing* will inform and support prescribers and that it will make an important contribution to improvements in both the quality and accessibility of patient care.

Dr June Crown CBE

Preface

The introduction of non-medical prescribing has meant that nurses and pharmacists have had to expand their practice and so acquire new knowledge and skills in a number of fields. This new knowledge has had to be applied to the many issues surrounding prescribing in the practice setting. There are currently few books available that provide these prescribers with information to help them in this role. As non-medical prescribing extends to include allied health professionals, the need for such information will increase. This book is aimed at those non-medical professions involved in prescribing medicines.

Chapter 1 provides a general overview of non-medical prescribing and describes the current education and training available for extended independent and supplementary prescribers. Chapters 2–5 examine non-medical prescribing within a multi-disciplinary team context, the different models of consultation that might be used by prescribers and the legal and ethical aspects surrounding prescribing. The psychology and sociology of prescribing, applied pharmacology and monitoring skills are explored in Chapters 6–8. Chapters 9–12 deal with medicines concordance, evidence-based prescribing, prescribing within a public health context and the calculation skills required by prescribers. The concluding chapter describes how independent and supplementary prescribing can be used by non-medical prescribers. The treatment management of patients with dermatological conditions are used as an example. It is hoped that insights gained from this chapter will be applicable to other practice settings.

Each chapter is fully referenced and where appropriate readers are offered suggestions for further reading and other information sources. We hope that this book will make a positive contribution in a very important aspect of patient care.

Molly Courtenay
Matt Griffiths
2004

Contributors

John Adams RGN, MA, MPhil
Academic Programme Leader, School of Health Studies, Homerton College,
Cambridge

Anne Baird RGN, A51 (Practice Nursing), MA Health Care Practice
(Nurse Practitioner)
Extended Formulary/Supplementary Nurse Prescriber, Nurse Practitioner/
Nurse Team Leader, Porter Brook Medical Centre, Sheffield
Associate Lecturer, Sheffield Hallam University

Polly Buchanan RGN, RM, ONC, DipN, BSc(Hons)
Consultant Nurse, Business Development, Galderma UK

Stephen Chapman BSc(Hons), PhD, Cert H Econ, FRSM, MRPharmS
Professor of Prescribing Studies, Department of Medicines Management,
Keele University

Michele Cossey B(Pharm), MRPharmS, MSc
Clinical Development Manager (Pharmacy & Prescribing) , North and East
Yorkshire and Northern Lincolnshire Workforce Development Confederation,
National Prescribing Centre Trainer, Visiting Lecturer University of York

Molly Courtenay PhD, MSc, BSc, CertEd, RGN, RNT
Reader in Prescribing and Medicines Management, School of Health and
Social Care, University of Reading, Joint Prescribing Adviser, Royal College
of Nursing

Alison Eggleton MSc, MEd, BSc, Dip(French) Open, MRPharmS
Addenbrooke's Hospital NHS Trust, Cambridge

Mark Gagan RN, RNT, PGDip Social Research
Lecturer in Adult Nursing, Bournemouth University

Trudy Granby RN, DN, MSc Clinical Nursing
Assistant Director, Non-medical Prescribing Support, National Prescribing Centre,
Withington Hospital, Manchester

Matt Griffiths RGN, A&E Cert, FAETC
Senior Lecturer, Prescribing, School of Health Studies, Homerton College,
Cambridge,
Joint Prescribing Adviser, Royal College of Nursing

Sue Latter BSc(Hons), PhD, RN, PGDipHV
Reader, School of Nursing and Midwifery, University of Southampton

Lesley Metcalfe RGN, RM, BSc(Hons)
Arrowe Park Hospital, Wirral, Merseyside

Sarah J O'Brien MB BS, FFPH, DTM&H
Consultant Epidemiologist, Health Protection Agency, Communicable Diseases
Surveillance Centre (CDSC), London

Barbara Stuttle CBE, RN, DN, MHM
Director of Integrated Care and Executive Nurse, Castle Point and Rochford PCT,
Rayleigh, Essex,
Chair, Association of Nurse Prescribing

Tom Walley MD, FRCP, MRCGP
Professor of Clinical Pharmacology, Department of Pharmacology and
Therapeutics, University of Liverpool

Paul Warburton RN, MSc, CertEd, ENB 125
Heart Failure Nurse Specialist, Countess of Chester Hospital, Chester

Trisha Weller MHS, RGN, NDN Cert, CPT, DPSCHN(PN)
Head of Quality Assurance, Asthma Module Leader, National Respiratory
Training Centre, Warwick

Robin Williams MSc, RMN, RGN, CPN Cert, Dip Nursing(London),
IHSM(Diploma)
Nurse Clinician and Honorary Lecturer, Department of Pharmacology and
Therapeutics, University of Liverpool

Chapter 1

Non-medical prescribing: an overview

Molly Courtenay and Matt Griffiths

In 1986, recommendations were made for nurses to take on the role of prescribing. The Cumberlege Report Neighbourhood Nursing: A Focus for Care (Department of Health and Social Security (DHSS), 1986) examined the care given to clients in their homes by district nurses (DNs) and health visitors (HVs). It was identified that some very complicated procedures had arisen around prescribing in the community and that nurses were wasting their time requesting prescriptions from the general practitioner (GP) for such items as wound dressings and ointments. The report suggested that patient care could be improved and resources used more effectively if community nurses were able to prescribe as part of their everyday nursing practice, from a limited list of items and simple agents agreed by the DHSS.

Following the publication of this report, the recommendations for prescribing and its implications were examined. An advisory group was set up by the Department of Health (DoH) to examine nurse prescribing (*Crown Report*, DoH, 1989). Dr June Crown was the Chair of this group.

The following is taken from the Crown Report:

> *Nurses in the community take a central role in caring for patients in their homes. Nurse are not, however, able to write prescriptions for the products that are needed for patient care, even when the nurse is effectively taking professional responsibility for some aspects of the management of the patient. However experienced or highly skilled in their own areas of practice, nurses must ask a doctor to write a prescription. It is well known that in practice a doctor often rubber-stamps a prescribing decision taken by a nurse. This can lead to a lack of clarity about professional responsibilities, and is demeaning to both nurses and doctors. There is wide agreement that action is now needed to align prescribing powers with professional responsibility.*
>
> DoH (1989)

The report made a number of recommendations involving the categories of items that nurses might prescribe, together with the circumstances under which they might be prescribed. It was recommended that:

> *Suitably qualified nurses working in the community should be able, in clearly defined circumstances, to prescribe from a limited list of items and to adjust the timing and dosage of medicines within a set protocol.*
>
> DoH (1989)

The Crown Report identified several groups of patients that would benefit from nurse prescribing. These patients included: patients with a catheter or a stoma, patients suffering with post-operative wounds and homeless families not registered with a GP. The Report also suggested that a number of other benefits would occur as a result of nurses adopting the role of prescriber. As well as improved patient care, this included improved use of both nurses' and patients' time and improved communication between team members arising as a result of a clarification of professional responsibilities (DoH, 1989).

During 1992, the primary legislation permitting nurses to prescribe a limited range of drugs was passed *(Medicinal Products: Prescribing by Nurses Act 1992)*. The necessary amendments were made to this Act in 1994 and a revised list of products available to the nurse prescriber was published in the Nurse Prescribers' Formulary (NPF) (NPF, 2003). In 1994, eight demonstration sites were set up in England for nurse prescribing. By the Spring of 2001, approximately 20,000 DNs and HVs were qualified independent prescribers and post-registration programmes for DNs and HVs included the necessary educational component qualifying nurses to prescribe.

The available research exploring independent nurse prescribing by DNs and HVs indicates that patients are as satisfied, and sometimes more satisfied with a nurse prescribing as they are with their GP. The quality of the relationship that the nurse has with the patient, the accessibility of the nurse and their approachability, the style of consultation and information provided, and the expertise of the nurse are attributes of nurse prescribing viewed positively by patients (Luker *et al.*, 1998). Nurse prescribing enables doctors and nurses to use their time more effectively and treatments are more conveniently provided (Brooks *et al.*, 2001). Time saving and convenience (with regard to not seeing a GP to supply a prescription) are benefits reported by nurses adopting the role of prescriber (Luker *et al.*, 1997). Furthermore, nurses are of the opinion that they provide the patient with better information about their treatment and have reported an increased sense of satisfaction, status and autonomy (Luker *et al.*, 1997; Rodden, 2001).

A further report by Crown, which reviewed the prescribing, supply and administration of medicines, was published in 1999 (DoH, 1999). The review recommended that prescribing authority should be extended to other groups of professionals with training and expertise in specialist areas. During 2001, support was given by the government for this extension (DoH, 2001). Funding was made available for other nurses, as well as those currently qualified to prescribe, to undergo the necessary training to enable them to prescribe from an extended formulary.

This formulary included:

- A number of specified Prescription-Only-Medicines (POMs), enabling nurses to prescribe for a number of conditions listed within four treatment areas, i.e. minor ailments, minor injuries, health promotion and palliative care.

- General Sales List (GSL) items, i.e. those that can be sold to the public without the supervision of a pharmacist, used to treat these conditions.

- Pharmacy (P) medicines, i.e. those products sold under the supervision of a pharmacist, used to treat these conditions.

During 2003, proposals by the Medicines and Healthcare Products Regulatory Agency (MHRA, 2003) to expand the Nurse Prescribers Extended Formulary (NPEF) were accepted and the NPEF was extended to include a number of additional conditions and medicines (NPF, 2003). The government also promised that the formulary would be further extended in 2004 to include medicines prescribable by nurses working in first contact and emergency care.

Further legislation was also passed by the Home Office in 2003, allowing nurses to prescribe a number of controlled drugs (CDs). These include:

1. Diazepam, lorazepam, midazolam (schedule 4 drugs) for use in palliative care.
2. Codeine phosphate, dihydrocodeine and co-phenotrope (schedule 5 drugs).

A number of other CDs, included in the proposals set out by the MHRA (2003), are expected to be added to the NPEF in 2004, following Home Office approval. These include pain relief in palliative care and diamorphine in coronary care.

EDUCATIONAL PREPARATION FOR EXTENDED PRESCRIBERS

An outline curriculum for the educational preparation for extended independent prescribing was produced by the English National Board (ENB) for Nursing and Midwifery in September 2001 (ENB, 2001). Following the closure of the ENB, the Nursing and Midwifery Council (NMC) have continued to apply the ENB's existing standards and guidance for the approval of higher education institutions (HEIs) with regards to registerable and recordable programmes (Letters; 8 November 2001; 21 March 2002).

The extended independent prescribing programme is 3–6 months in length and includes 25 taught days, additional self-directed study, plus 12 days learning in practice with a medical mentor. The areas of study included within the prescribing module (ENB, 2001) are those general concepts that underpin prescribing. Topics include:

- Consultation, decision-making and therapy including referral
- Influences on and psychology of prescribing
- Prescribing in a team context
- Clinical pharmacology including the effects of co-morbidity
- Evidenced-based practice and clinical governance in relation to nurse prescribing
- Legal, policy and ethical aspects
- Professional accountability and responsibility
- Prescribing in the public health context.

SUPPLEMENTARY PRESCRIBING

The introduction of a new form of prescribing for professions allied to medicine was suggested in 1999 (DoH, 1999). It was proposed that this new form of prescribing, i.e. 'dependent' prescribing would take place after a diagnosis had been made by a doctor and a Clinical Management Plan (CMP) drawn up for the patient. The term 'dependent' prescribing, has since been superseded by 'supplementary prescribing'.

Supplementary prescribing is *a voluntary prescribing partnership between an independent prescriber (doctor) and a supplementary prescriber (SP) (nurse or pharmacist, to implement an agreed patient-specific CMP with the patient's agreement* (DoH, 2002). Patients with long-term medical conditions such as asthma, diabetes or coronary heart disease, or those with long-term health needs such as anti-coagulation therapy are most likely to benefit from this type of prescribing.

Unlike independent prescribing, there are no legal restrictions on the clinical conditions for which SPs are able to prescribe. Nurses adopting the role of SP will be able to prescribe:

- All GSL and P medicines, appliances and devices, foods and other borderline substances approved by the Advisory Committee on Borderline Substances.

- All POMs with the current exception of CDs – the Home Office are currently deliberating on a consultation to potentially instigate changes in the law to make this possible.

- 'Off-label' medicines (medicines for use outside their licensed indications), 'black triangle' drugs and drugs marked 'less suitable for prescribing' in the British National Formulary (BNF).

- Unlicensed drugs may only be prescribed if they are part of a clinical trial with a clinical trial certificate or exemption (this may change following proposals set out by the MHRA (2004) enabling SP to prescribe unlicensed medicines).

Training for supplementary prescribing was introduced in 2003 for nurses and pharmacists. However, the government has promised that other professions allied to medicine will be able to prescribe as of 2004.

Training for supplementary prescribing is based on that for extended independent prescribing. For nurses, the taught element of the course is 26/27 days, of which a substantial proportion is face-to-face contact time, although, other ways of learning, such as open and distance learning (DL) formats, might be used. Students are also required to undertake additional self-directed learning and 12/13 days learning in practice with a medical prescriber.

Training for extended independent prescribing is combined with that for SP in the majority of HEIs. The Royal Pharmaceutical Society of Great Britain (RPSGB), responsible for validating SP programmes for pharmacists has acknowledged that as between 60% and 70% of the SP curriculum will be common to both nurses and pharmacists, institutions running the SP curriculum for nurses provide an ideal opportunity for shared learning. Therefore, a number of HEIs run the combined extended independent/supplementary prescribing programme for nurses and pharmacists. Nurses qualify as both extended independent and SPs upon successful completion of the course and pharmacists qualify as SPs.

In England, the extended independent prescribing module attracts 20 credit accumulation and transfer scheme (CATS) points at level 3. The combined extended

SP programme awards an additional 10 credit accumulation and transfer scheme (CATS) points, i.e. a total of 30 CATS points. This is in contrast to regions with devolved governments (e.g. Northern Ireland). In these instances, HEIs are able to award a greater number of credits. One such institution in Northern Ireland is currently awarding 60 CATS points to nurses undergoing prescribing preparation.

Entry requirements for extended independent and SP programmes include:

- Registration with the NMC as a first level Nurse or Midwife or, for pharmacists, current registration with the RPSGB and/or the Pharmaceutical Society of Northern Ireland (PSNI).
- The ability to study at level 3.
- At least 3 year's post-registration clinical nursing experience (or part-time equivalent). For pharmacists, the level of relevant knowledge and expertise is dependent upon the nature of their practice and the length of their experience.
- Have a medical prescriber willing to contribute to the students 12/13 days learning in practice (including the assessment process), and supervised prescribe post-qualifying.
- Agreement by their employing organisation to undertake the programme, a period of supervised practice, and continuing professional development (CPD).
- Commitment by their employer to enable access to prescribing budgets and other necessary arrangements for prescribing in practice.
- Occupy a post in which they are expected to prescribe (RPSGB, 2003; ENB, 2001).

For further discussion of supplementary prescribing see Chapter 2.

CONCLUSION

Until recently, the development of non-medical prescribing has been slow. It was first considered by the government for nurses in 1986. However, as of 2001, the introduction of extended independent and SP has been considered for other healthcare professionals (including other 1st level nurses as well as those with a DN/HV qualification).

Training for independent extended prescribing for nurses commenced in 2002. Nurses are now able to prescribe independently from a list of medicines (including CDs) for an array of conditions and the government has promised that the NPEF will be further extended to include prescribing in first contact and emergency care. Independent prescribing for pharmacists is currently under consideration.

Training for supplementary prescribing was introduced for nurses and pharmacists in 2003. SPs can prescribe from virtually the whole of the BNF and may include CDs as of 2004. Other groups of healthcare professionals are to be considered by the government for prescribing this year. DoH funding for extended independent and supplementary prescribing has been extended until 2005/2006 and the government aims to train 10,000 nurses and 1000 pharmacists during this period.

References

Brooks N, Otway C, Rashid C, Kilty E, Maggs C (2001). The patients' view: the benefits and limitations of nurse prescribing. *British Journal of Community Nursing* **6(7)**: 342–348.

DHSS (1986). *Neighbourhood Nursing: A Focus for Care (Cumberlege Report)*. London: HMSO.

DoH (1989). *Report of the Advisory Group on Nurse Prescribing (Crown Report)*. London: DoH.

DoH (1999). *Review of Prescribing, Supply and Administration of Medicines (Crown Report)*. London: DoH.

DoH (2001). *Patients to Get Quicker Access to Medicines (Press Release)*. London: DoH.

DoH (2002). *Supplementary Prescribing*. London: DoH.

English National Board for Nursing, Midwifery & Health Visiting (2001). *Education Policy Letter 2001/01/TL* of September 2001.

Luker KA, Austin L, Hogg C, Ferguson B, Smith K (1998). Nurse–patient relationships: the context of nurse prescribing. *Journal of Advanced Nursing* **28(2)**: 235–242.

Luker K, Austin L, Ferguson B, Smith K (1997). Nurse prescribing: the views of nurses and other healthcare professionals. *British Journal of Community Health Nursing* **2**: 69–74.

MHRA (2003). *Consultation Document MLX293, NPEF.*

MHRA (2004). Supplementary prescribing: use of unlicensed medicines, reformulation of licensed products and preparations made from active pharmaceutical ingredients and excipients.

NPF (2003–2005). British Medical Association, Royal Pharmaceutical Society of Great Britain. In association with Community Practitioners' and Health Visitors' Association, Royal College of Nursing.

Rodden C (2001). Nurse prescribing: views on autonomy and independence. *British Journal of Community Nursing* **6(7)**: 350–355.

RPSGB (2003). Outline curriculum for training programmes to prepare pharmacist supplementary prescribers. http://www.rpsgb.org.uk

Chapter 2

Non-medical prescribing in a multidisciplinary team context

Barbara Stuttle

The demands by patients for a more streamlined, accessible and flexible service (Department of Health (DoH), 2000), demands for a high quality accountable service and for roles which extend beyond traditional boundaries, acknowledging the range of knowledge and skills held by practitioners and offering them the opportunity to achieve their full potential (DoH, 2001; 2002), has meant that the roles of healthcare professionals have changed dramatically over recent years. These changes have placed a great emphasis on teamwork and multiprofessional co-operation.

The success of non-medical prescribing is dependent upon the contributions from a number of practitioners, including specialist nurses, pharmacists and doctors and the ability of these professionals to work together as a team. This chapter examines the key issues that need to be considered by healthcare professionals if non-medical prescribing is to be implemented effectively. It commences with an exploration of teamwork and then moves on to discuss clinical governance. Communication, sharing information, and supplementary prescribing are then examined.

TEAMWORK

In order to work effectively as a team, a number of key elements are required. These include:

- effective verbal and written communication;

- enabling and encouraging supervision;

- collaboration and common goals;

- valuing the contributions of team members and matching team roles to ability;

- a culture that encourages team members to seek help;

- team structure (Vincent *et al.*, 1998).

Underpinning each of the above elements is the need for team members to have a clear understanding of one another's roles. As non-medical prescribing has changed the role boundaries of professions allied to medicine, so the roles and relationships between healthcare professionals have changed. For example, the nurse adopting the role of prescriber affects the role of the pharmacist. The conversations surrounding medicines that once took place between the pharmacist and the doctor, now take place between the pharmacist, doctor and the nurse.

Conversely, it is important that the nurse is aware of the support the pharmacist is able to provide. This support will vary depending upon the environment within which the pharmacist works. If the pharmacist is working in a hospital setting and as a member of the ward team, they will have greater information about the patient's conditions and specific problems. The role of the pharmacist is therefore enhanced. As well as the interpretation of prescriptions, checking drug dosage levels, and monitoring prescriptions for possible drug interactions, they may well be able to advise colleagues on a number of topics in relation to drug therapy, undertake medication reviews, discharge planning, education and training (Downie et al., 2003). Furthermore, with the introduction of supplementary prescribing, pharmacists may well be leading clinics such as anticoagulation or pain control clinics and so be able to provide the nurse with a greater wealth of information.

Another area in which confusion may occur, if roles are not fully understood, is level of competency. For example, the ability of a nurse to prescribe, means that they are able to carry out a complete episode of care. However, not all nurses within a team are qualified to prescribe. Therefore, there may be a lack of consistency or continuity of care if other non-nurse prescribers care for the patient. Unless these different levels of competency with regards to prescribing are understood between team members, this could result in inequity of service and confusion for the patient.

The advent of non-medical prescribing, has therefore emphasised the need to clarify the activity of team members, i.e. those activities common to some professions, and those specific to the role of one discipline only. It has been suggested that without this clarity, team members might drift towards common ground and some areas of practice could become neglected (McCray, 2002).

The core values of multidisciplinary work have been described as trust and sharing (Loxley, 1997). An essential component of these values is that trust and sharing are a two-way process. Not only does the team rely on the individual's commitment to the task, but also, members must take on the teams' belief in one's self and meet their expectations. If members of the team are to trust one another and share their experiences, confidence and a clear understanding of one's own professional role is essential (Loxley, 1997).

For example, nurses have traditionally been seen as semi-autonomous practitioners working within the guidelines set by doctors. Medical staff have been seen as those making autonomous decisions and advising on practice. Some professions allied to medicine, for example physiotherapists, although practising autonomously, work primarily on an individual basis with clients. It is suggested by McCray (2002) that power and status, as a result of these differences, may well become an issue and influence trust and sharing when working together in a team. Doctors may well find it difficult to take advice from some healthcare professionals. By contrast, nurses may not feel confident enough to provide advice in relation to their own area of practice.

CLINICAL GOVERNANCE

Clinical governance has been defined as:

A framework through which National Health Services (NHS) organisations are accountable for continually improving the quality of their services and safeguarding high standards of care by creating an environment to which excellence in clinical care will flourish.

Scally and Donaldson (1998)

Clinical governance has been responsible for bringing professionals together as a multiprofessional team, to collaborate and learn from each other. This has meant moving away from a culture of self-protection and blame, to one where self-regulation and learning through experience is valued (Jasper, 2002). By working together and reflecting on the skills and knowledge of team members, the opportunities for progress and improvement in patient care are immense. The Bristol Royal Infirmary Inquiry (doh.gov.uk/bristolinquiry) and Victoria Climbie (http://www.victoria-climbie-inquiry.org.uk/finreport/finreport.htm) provide examples of where teamwork and communication have broken down. Recommendations from these reports focus on team working, communication, sharing information and joint learning.

Drug therapy is becoming increasingly complex. Many patients receive multiple drugs and therefore, the possibility of error while administering medicines is large. An error that involves the administration of a drug can be a disaster for the patient. Drug administration generally involves several members of the multidisciplinary team and will include a chain of events involving several people, i.e. the manufacturers, distributors, pharmacists, prescribers, hospital managers, and the patients. A number of errors that may occur at each level have been identified by Downie *et al.* (2003). These include:

- Prescribers error:
  - Poor handwriting
  - Abbreviations
  - Confusion of product names that look similar
  - Omission of essential information

- Pharmacist error:
  - Errors in labelling medicines
  - The supply of medicines to wards without information on the actions, dose and use of the product
  - The lack of withdrawal of a product due to fault (i.e. there is a need for rapid communication from pharmaceutical staff to ward staff)
  - Lack of information about a product that is part of a clinical trial: if information is not supplied to ward staff involved in the trial, the product may not be used safely

- Error by the nurse administering the medicine:
  - Misinterpretation of the prescription
  - Selection of the incorrect medicine to be administered
  - Inaccurate record of administration

- Error by the nurse manager:
  - Lack of up-to-date drug information (i.e. British National Formulary (BNF) and local formularies unavailable)
  - No clear lines of communication with clinical pharmacists and Medicines Information Service
  - Inappropriate staff members administering medicines
  - Inaccurate and illegible records regarding the drugs administered
  - Unsafe storage of medicines
  - Lack of withdrawal of medicines when no longer required
  - No consideration to timing and number of medicine rounds
  - Prescribing and recording documents not of the required standard and inappropriate for the area of practice
  - Procedures used in the event of a drug error seen as a deterrent by nurses, i.e. a 'blame' culture
  - An absence of a multidisciplinary drug and therapeutics committee to review medicines management issues
  - Level of risk not assessed (i.e. some drugs more complicated to administer than others)

- Patient error:
  - Lack of co-operation by the patient in order to achieve therapeutic benefits of the drug
  - The rejection of treatment by the patient as a result of a lack of understanding (by the patient) about the drug therapy.

Clinical governance is a useful tool that can be used by the multidisciplinary team to maintain and improve the quality of non-medical prescribing and demonstrate that prescribing practice is in the best interest of the patient. It should ensure that each member of the prescribing team (i.e. doctor, nurse and pharmacist) recognise their role in providing high quality patient care, and how the team can work together to improve prescribing standards.

Regular team meetings provide a forum in which members of the multidisciplinary team can work together to achieve common goals, and develop standards of care and protocols for prescribing. Within these meetings, awareness needs to be raised with regards to such systems as the Yellow Card Scheme for the spontaneous reporting of suspected adverse drug reactions by doctors, dentists, pharmacists, coroners and nurses (http://medicines.mhra.gov.uk/) and the National Patient Safety Agency (NPSA), for reporting drug errors (http://www.npsa.nhs.uk/). The NPSA hope that by promoting a fair and open culture in the NHS, staff will be encouraged to report incidents and so learn from any problems that affect the safety of patients. If team meetings raise staff awareness of the NPSA and errors are discussed, this will enable individuals to reflect and learn from mistake and to take the appropriate action to prevent it happening again. There will be a move away from a 'blame' culture, and patient safety will be increased.

Once standards of care have been set and implemented by members of the multiprofessional team, the team will be able to undertake periodic audits of prescribing practice. The outcome of these audits can be used to identify areas of prescribing practice that require improvement, and also the education and training needs of individuals. All healthcare professionals have a responsibility for their individual professional development and maintenance of prescribing knowledge. By working as a multiprofessional team, the needs of individuals can be identified, education and training programmes accessed, and learning shared across professional boundaries.

COMMUNICATION AND SHARING INFORMATION

The sharing of accurate information between multidisciplinary team members is vitally important. It was highlighted by the Crown Report (DoH, 1989) that good communication between health professionals and patients, and between different professionals, is essential for high quality healthcare.

Good record keeping in relation to prescribing is essential and provides an efficient method of communication and dissemination of information between members of the multidisciplinary team. The healthcare record is a tool for communication within the team. It should provide clear evidence of the care planned, the decisions made, the care delivered and the information shared.

The prescription details, together with other details of the consultation with the patient, should be entered into the patient's record. The record should clearly indicate the date, the name of the prescriber, the name of the items prescribed and the quantity prescribed (or dose, frequency and treatment duration) at the time of generating the prescription. Where nurses hold separate nursing records, they have a responsibility to ensure this information is entered into the medical record as soon as possible and preferably contemporaneously. All health professionals qualified to prescribe should have access to the relevant patient records. Ideally, these records should be shared between team members.

SUPPLEMENTARY PRESCRIBING AND TEAMWORK

Supplementary prescribing is described in Chapter 1. The information outlined below can be found at http://www.dh.gov.uk/PolicyAndGuidance/Medicines PharmacyAndIndustryServices/Prescriptions/SupplementaryPrescribing/fs/en. The nature of Supplementary prescribing heightens the need for good teamwork. The patient, independent prescriber (IP) and supplementary prescriber (SP) are required to work in partnership to develop the Clinical Management Plan (CMP) (see Figures 2.1 and 2.2). The IP is responsible for the diagnosis and setting the parameters of the CMP, although they need not personally draw it up. The principle underlying the concept of supplementary prescribing must be explained in advance to the patient by the IP or the SP and their agreement should be obtained. The IP and the SP must agree and sign the CMP.

It should also be clear from information recorded on the CMP as to when the plan will be reviewed by the IP. Supplementary prescribing must be supported by a regular clinical review of the patient's progress by the assessing clinician (the IP), at predetermined intervals appropriate to the patient's condition and the medicines to be prescribed. This may be a joint review by both the independent and SP. Where this is not possible, the IP should review the patient, and subsequently discuss the future management of the patient's condition(s) with the SP. The intervals should normally be no longer than one year.

Name of patient:	Patient medication sensitivities/allergies:
Patient identification e.g. ID number, date of birth:	

IP(s):	SP(s):
Condition(s) to be treated:	Aim of treatment:

Medicines that may be prescribed by SP:

Preparation	Indication	Dose schedule	Specific indications for referral back to the IP

Guidelines or protocols supporting Clinical management plan:

Frequency of review and monitoring by:

SP:	SP and IP:

Process for reporting ADRs:

Shared record to be used by IP and SP:

Agreed by IP(s):	Date	Agreed by SP(s):	Date	Date agreed with patient/carer

Figure 2.1 The CMP (for teams that have full co-terminus access to patient records) (http://www.dh.gov.uk/PolicyAndGuidance/MedicinesPharmacyAnd IndustryServices/Prescriptions/SupplementaryPrescribing/fs/en)

Name of patient:	Patient medication sensitivities/allergies:
Patient identification e.g. ID number, date of birth:	
Current medication:	Medical history:
IP(s): Contact details: [tel/email/address]	SP(s): Contact details: [tel/email/address]
Condition(s) to be treated:	Aim of treatment:

Medicines that may be prescribed by SP:			
Preparation	Indication	Dose schedule	Specific indications for referral back to the IP

Guidelines or protocols supporting Clinical management plan:	
Frequency of review and monitoring by:	
SP:	SP and IP:
Process for reporting ADRs:	
Shared record to be used by IP and SP:	

Agreed by IP(s):	Date	Agreed by SP(s):	Date	Date agreed with patient/carer

Figure 2.2 CMP (for teams where the SP does not have co-terminus access to the medical record) (http://www.dh.gov.uk/PolicyAndGuidance/Medicines PharmacyAndIndustryServices/Prescriptions/SupplementaryPrescribing/fs/en)

Both prescribers must record their agreement to the continuing or amended CMP, and the patient's agreement to the continuation of the supplementary prescribing arrangement, in order for the CMP to remain valid. They should set a new review date. Prescribing by the SP should not continue after the date of review without a recorded agreement to the next phase of the CMP.

Discontinuation of supplementary prescribing is at the discretion of the IP. However, this mode of prescribing can be discontinued at the request of the SP or the patient. Furthermore, where there is a sole IP and he or she is replaced for whatever reason, the CMP must be reviewed by their successor.

In order for effective implementation of supplementary prescribing, the following factors are important:

- It must be simple, i.e. the CMP should not duplicate information already in the shared records.

- The CMP need only make a reference to the appropriate guideline for the treatment of a condition. There is no need to produce lists of medicines.

- Supplementary prescribing must be flexible. The IP and SP will need to work differently in different settings. For example, if the IP and SP are not in close contact, shared electronic records might be required. There may also be a need for team partnerships, i.e. the SP may need to form a partnership with more than one IP.

CONCLUSION

If non-medical prescribing is to be a success, it is important that those healthcare professionals involved in prescribing develop good relationships with one another. This will lead to trust, confidence, respect, the sharing of information, and a clear understanding on one another's role. This will enable individuals to work together effectively as a team.

Clinical governance is a useful tool that should be used by the multiprofessional team in order to maintain and improve the quality of non-medical prescribing; should ensure that each member of the team recognises their role in providing a high quality of patient care, and how the team can work together to improve standards.

References

DoH (2002). *Liberating the Talents*. The Stationery Office: London.

DoH (2001). *Essence of Care*. DoH: London.

DoH (2000). *A Health Service of All the Talents: Developing the NHS Workforce*. DoH: London.

DoH (1989). *Report of the Advisory Group on Nurse Prescribing (Crown Report)*. London: DoH.

Downie G, Mackenzie J, Williams A (2003). *Pharmacology and Medicines Management for Nurses* 3rd edn. London: Churchill Livingstone.

http://medicines.mhra.gov.uk/

http://www.dh.gov.uk/PolicyAndGuidance/MedicinesPharmacyAndIndustry
Services/Prescriptions/SupplementaryPrescribing/fs/en

http://www.npsa.nhs.uk

Jasper M (2002). Challenges to professional practice In: *Foundations of Nursing Practice* (Hogston, R and Simpson, P). Basingstoke: Palgrave Macmillan.

Loxley A (1997). *Collaboration in Health and Welfare*. London: Jessica Kingsley.

McCray J (2002). Nursing practice in an interprofessional context In: *Foundations of Nursing Practice* (Hogston, R and Simpson, P). Basingstoke: Palgrave Macmillan.

Scally G, Donaldson LJ (1998). Clinical governance and the drive for quality improvement in the new NHS in England. *British Medical Journal* **317**: 61–65.

Vincent CA, Adams S, Stanhope N (1998). A framework for the analysis of risk and safety in medicines. *British Medical Journal* **316**: 1154–1157.

Chapter 3

Consultation skills and decision making

Anne Baird

INTRODUCTION

Much of the research on the consultation has developed from the desire of general practice to carve out for itself a specific body of expertise distinct from hospital medicine (Drucquer and Hutchinson, 2000). As a result, while there is a considerable amount of literature relating to general practice, as practised by the General Practitioner (GP), there is little on consultation by nurses and other health professionals, and little on consultations in secondary care. This chapter will endeavour to introduce to the reader some of the key texts on consultation models and communication skills, and discuss their relevance for non-medical prescribers. Patients' health beliefs will be briefly explored, as will the literature comparing the outcomes of consultations by doctors and other health professionals. Decision-making strategies and diagnosis will be looked at, with a brief overview of computer decision support in the consultation. A chapter such as this can only hope to give a brief synopsis of these issues, and it is hoped that the reader will use the reference list to follow up areas of particular interest in more detail.

CONSULTATION MODELS

The concept of nurses or pharmacists undertaking a consultation is relatively new. Whilst the consultation will for many prescribers form the basis of the interaction during which they prescribe, this will not be the case for all: consider ward based nurses and pharmacists, and nurses working in the patient's home. However, for practitioners working in all of these settings, many of the concepts discussed will be of relevance. It is interesting to note that whilst GP registrars are extensively trained and heavily assessed in consultation skills, other practitioners new to consulting may be given little or no support in gaining these skills. While they are able to draw on the communication skills they have always made use of, applying these within a different context can bring difficulties. The emphasis given to the consultation in the prescribing course will provide a valuable opportunity for many nurses and pharmacists to examine and improve their skills in this area.

So, what are consultation models and do they have any practical applications? The best-known models, which are discussed below, can be described as either normative (what should happen in a consultation) or descriptive (what does happen in a consultation).

Byrne and Long (1976)

One of the first examples of a descriptive model is that of Byrne and Long (1976), which is based on an analysis of over 2000 recorded consultations. They identified six phases to the consultation:

- Phase I   The doctor establishes a relationship with the patient

- Phase II   The doctor attempts to discover, or does discover, the reason for the patient's attendance

- Phase III   The doctor conducts a verbal or physical examination or both

- Phase IV   The doctor, or the doctor and the patient, or the patient (in that order of probability) consider the condition

- Phase V   The doctor, and occasionally the patient, detail further treatment or further investigation

- Phase VI   The consultation is terminated, usually by the doctor

- Phase VII   The 'parting shot'.

In reality, consultations rarely unfold in such a logical manner, though all phases are likely to occur at some stage (including, possibly, the 'parting shot' when the patient reveals the real reason for their attendance just as they are about to leave!). Byre and Long (1976) noted that, unsurprisingly, consultations are likely to go wrong if there are shortcomings in phase II (there is a failure to discover the reason for attending) or phase IV (there is a failure to adequately consider the implications of the problem). They also noted that, on average, doctors interrupted patients within 18 seconds of the start of the consultation!

Stott and Davies (1979)

Stott and Davies' model identified 4 areas that could potentially be explored within each consultation.

These are as follows:

- Management of the presenting problem. This is key, and if not dealt with, the patient is unlikely to be receptive to any other activities.

- Modification of help seeking behaviours. This could include, for example, a discussion on how to manage a sore throat at home in the future.

- Review of long-term problems, for example, blood pressure check.

- Opportunistic health promotion, for example, mentioning overdue cervical cytology or a discussion of smoking cessation.

Pendleton et al. (1984)

Pendleton *et al.* are best known for their discussion of the patient's ideas, concerns and expectations, and the concept of a patient-centred, rather than a doctor-centred, consultation. They detail seven tasks of the consultation. By now, similar themes are beginning to emerge from each of the models.

1. To define the reason for attendance, including:
   - The nature/history of the problem
   - Aetiology
   - Patients ideas, concerns and expectations
   - The effects of the problem

2. To consider other problems
   - Continuing problems
   - Risk factors

3. With the patient, to chose an appropriate action for each problem

4. To achieve a shared understanding of the problem with the patient

5. To involve the patient in the management and encourage him to accept appropriate responsibility

6. To use time and resources appropriately

7. To establish and maintain a relationship.

This model is one in which the practitioner works in partnership with the patient to find a solution satisfactory to both. For example, a mother bringing her child to surgery with a possible ear infection may believe that antibiotics are necessary, as they have previously been prescribed. Furthermore, she may believe that she would be negligent not to bring the child. Or the manager consulting with a sore throat may be anxious that he will be unable to deliver an important presentation next week. If the practitioner is able to acknowledge the importance to the patient of these concerns, it is more likely that a solution acceptable to both parties will be reached.

Factors 6 and 7 deal with concerns outwith the immediate consultation, but none the less important. An awareness of the finite nature of resources (e.g. time or money), and wisdom in their use, is essential for the well-being of the practitioner as well as for the patient. The establishing of a relationship, either for the duration of the consultation or which may in be ongoing for many years is also important for patient and practitioner satisfaction.

Neighbour (1987)
Roger Neighbour, in his most readable book, builds on the other models in his view of the consultation as a journey with 'checkpoints' along the way.

- *Connecting*: This first checkpoint is to do with establishing a relationship and building a rapport with the patient, and is identified by Neighbour as the first essential task of the consultation.

- *Summarising*: The second checkpoint includes taking a history, summarising the problem and reflecting it back to the patient to ensure there are no misunderstandings. It also involves considering the patient's ideas, concerns and expectations.

- *Handing over*: By this time, the practitioner will have brought the consultation to a point where the patient and the practitioner's agendas have been agreed and dealt with, and a management plan developed.

- *Safety netting*: This involves acknowledging that things may not turn out as planned, and ensuring that the patient knows what to do should this happen. It may involve sharing with the patient some of the other possible diagnoses and outcomes. For example, the patient with asthma could be advised to increase their bronchodilator inhaler, but to monitor their peak flows and to return if their peak flow continues to fall.

- *Housekeeping*: This is where the practitioner looks to themselves and their response to the consultation. It may involve having a brief chat with a colleague, a coffee, or merely acknowledging to oneself the effect a particular consultation has had.

Calgary–Cambridge model (1998)

More recently, Silverman, Kurtz and Draper have explored the consultation in considerable depth, through an approach that has become known as the Calgary–Cambridge model (so named because of its origins in the University of Calgary, Canada and the University of Cambridge, UK). They build upon the body of knowledge referred to in other well-known models. An outline plan of their model is described below, but readers are advised to consult the book for a more detailed study of their method.

1. Initiating the session
   - Establishing initial rapport
   - Involving the patient

2. Gathering information
   - Exploration of problems
   - Understanding the patients perspective
   - Providing structure to the consultation

3. Building the relationship
   - Developing rapport
   - Involving the patient

4. Explanation and planning
   - Providing the correct amount and type of information
   - Aiding accurate recall and understanding
   - Achieving a shared understanding
   - Planning – shared decision-making

5. Closing the session.

Silverman *et al.*'s work builds on the strong body of research into the consultation that precedes it, some of which has been discussed above. Again, similar themes are explored. The concept of the patient's agenda is prominent, whilst the value of providing structure to the consultation is stressed. It can be reassuring to realise that a patient-centred consultation does not mean that the practitioner abdicates all responsibility to the patient. Rather, both patient and practitioner will feel more secure if the practitioner is able to give some structure and direction to the consultation, whilst addressing the patient's concerns.

Silverman *et al.* also address specifically the issue of closing the session, something which nurses may find difficult, possibly because of the perception of many patients that nurses are more approachable and have more time than the doctor. Suggestions include agreeing on specific follow up and setting another appointment. Tate (2003) goes a step further in suggesting that standing up and holding the door open may be required! Personally, I have sometimes found it necessary to help particularly garrulous patients into their coats and gently guide them through the door!

COMMUNICATION SKILLS

Consultation models are helpful but without the use of appropriate skills on the part of the practitioner, they remain sterile. Much of the literature on consultation models also discusses the skills needed for an effective consultation. It has been shown that good communication skills on the part of the practitioner greatly affect the outcome of the consultation. Maguire and Pitceathly (2002) suggest that doctors with good consultation skills identify patients' problems more accurately. Patients are more satisfied with the care they receive, and leave the consultation with a better understanding of their problems, proposed investigations and treatment options. They are more likely to adhere to treatment and lifestyle changes, and distress and anxiety are lessened. An added bonus would appear to be increased well-being and satisfaction for the practitioner.

Communication skills are included in nurse's core training, but this does not mean that they can afford to be complacent. Chant (2002), in a literature review, has suggested that this training may at times be lacking and that there is a wide variation in the quality of nurse/patient communication. Whilst Bond *et al.* (1999) found that trainee nurse practitioners rated uniformly high in consultation skills, another study by Greco and Powel (2002) suggests that although this is generally true, it is by no means always the case.

Which communication skills are required for an effective consultation? What follows is of necessity a brief overview; readers are directed to more comprehensive texts for a more thorough examination of the topic. Silvermann and Kurtz (1998) have identified a total of 72 skills which can be used within the consultation, and most of the literature on consultation models also examines the necessary skills.

The consultation skills needed by the nurse prescriber are no different to those used in other aspects of nursing practice. An appropriate environment, i.e. one which supports privacy and confidentiality, is important (While, 2002), and may pose particular challenges for ward based prescribers and those working in the patient's home. Strategies to support the patient in telling their story include open and closed questioning, active listening and the appropriate use of eye contact and other body language. The recent interest in narrative based medicine (Launer, 2002), where the telling of the patient's story is central to the consultation, draws heavily upon the skills used in family therapy.

Central to the success of the consultation is the ability of the practitioner to identify what the patient hopes to get out of the consultation – i.e. their ideas, concerns and expectations (Pendleton, 1984). Research has shown that many patients find it difficult to voice their true concerns (Barry *et al.*, 2000), leading the authors to suggest that patients are not 'fully present' in the consultation. This failure in communication may contribute to inappropriate prescribing decisions; for example, the doctor may prescribe and the patient may take medicine, both just for the sake of the relationship (Britten, 2000). There has been a tendency for doctors to assume that patients consult for the sake of a prescription, whereas on many occasions, they may prefer advice or simply be seeking reassurance (Barry *et al.*, 2000; Britten *et al.*, 2000). Nurse–patient consultations have to some extent been free of this preconception until recently, and nurse prescribers will need to take care to ensure that they continue to reserve the prescription only for those situations where it is genuinely required.

THE PATIENT'S HEALTH BELIEFS

Stewart and Roter (1989) have discussed in their disease-illness model an analysis of the different perspective of patient and practitioner for the sickness they are experiencing. According to this model, 'disease' is the cause of sickness in terms of pathophysiology, whilst 'illness' is the patient's unique experience of sickness. Patients can experience illness but have no disease; for example, the many patients who present in general practice complaining of tiredness, for which no organic cause can be found. Similarly, patients may have a disease without experiencing illness, for example, the patient with hypertension is likely to feel completely well. Similar diseases may cause a widely varying illness experience in different individuals, due to their concerns, expectation, support systems and previous experiences (Silverman, 1998). This theory goes some way to explain why one individual may consult for an episode of ill health (e.g. a sore throat) whereas another is quite happy to let nature take its course. Traditionally, doctors have confined themselves seeking out underlying disease, but this perspective is narrower than that of the patient and may lead to an unsatisfactory conclusion.

Patients' illness experience depends to a great extent upon their perspective on their health. Rotter's locus of control theory and Rosenstock's health belief model (Kemm and Close, 1995) go some way to explaining why patients have such widely varying health experiences, and are discussed briefly below.

Many readers will be familiar with the concept of the locus of control (Rotter, 1954), which is concerned with the extent to which an individual feels able to influence and control their own life.

According to this theory, people's health beliefs fall into three broad categories:

- *Internal locus of control*: These individuals tend to believe that they are responsible for their own health and that what happens to them is the result of their own actions. They will tend to like explanations and discussion, and will want to be involved in decision-making about their health.

- *External locus of control*: Those with an external locus of control tend to have a fatalistic attitude to life and health, and will be reluctant to make changes as they believe that their future is mapped out and there is nothing to be done about it.

- *The powerful other*: These people will tend to see the responsibility for their health as lying with other people, such as health professionals. They will be reluctant to take responsibility for their own health and are most happy with an authoritarian approach.

Of course, these are broad categories, and most people will lie somewhere along the continuum. They may well espouse different belief systems for different areas of their lives. Tate (2003) suggests that an awareness of where an individual's locus of control lies can help the practitioner to adopt the most appropriate skills.

Another well-known model is Rosenstock's health belief model (1974). He suggests that an individual's motivation to take action is dependent upon four factors:

- *Perceived vulnerability*: For example, those who believe that they are likely to develop lung cancer are more likely to heed advice to stop smoking that those who do not believe that they are at risk.

- *Perceived seriousness*: Hypertension may not be regarded as a serious condition to some people, as it does not cause them to feel unwell. However, to the woman who has just lost her mother to a stroke it may seem very serious.

- *Perceived benefits*: People will weigh up the advantages and disadvantages of a particular course of action. To the individual with high blood pressure, the side-effects of the treatment may seem to outweigh any supposed benefit.

- *Perceived barriers*: The various barriers a person would need to overcome to go along with the suggested course of action, including physical, psychological and financial. To the person unconvinced of the need to treat high blood pressure, the financial implications of the prescription charge may prove to be the final disincentive.

An awareness of these factors may help the practitioner to understand the patient's particular anxieties and to tailor their interventions accordingly.

CONSULTATIONS WITH NURSES

Much of the literature comparing consultations by nurses and doctors examines the outcomes of the consultation, rather than the process of consulting. Most of it also relates to a general practice setting, in particular that of nurses running minor illness/first point of contact services. The outcomes do, however, shed some light on the consulting style favoured by nurses, suggesting that it would tend to be patient- rather than practitioner-centred.

Reveley (1998) in an analysis of the role of the triage nurse in general practice, suggests that patients value the caring and supportive aspects of consulting with a nurse, the length of time they have with the nurse, and the accessibility of the nurse. Many other studies (Horrocks *et al.*, 2002; Shum *et al.*, 2000; Kinnersley, 2000) have found greater patient satisfaction with nurse consultation than with GP consultations (although patients report high levels of satisfaction with both). Importantly, they also found no significant difference in other health outcomes – as Tate (2003) pointed out, patient satisfaction is a blunt (if popular) tool with which to measure the success of the consultation. Many patients will be satisfied if they get what they want, even if this does not necessarily represent best clinical practice.

Most of these studies found that consultations with nurses were slightly longer; that nurses gave more information to patients; and that they offered more advice on self-care and self-management. Interestingly, Kinnersley (2000) observed that although nurses gave more advice on self-care, a similar number of patients consulting with the nurse as with the doctor said they would consult again with the same condition. Kinnersley (2000) suggests that this may be because prescribing rates between the doctors and nurses were similar, validating the patient's decision to seek help rather than self-manage.

Most, if not all, of these studies observe that consultations with nurses are longer than consultations with doctors, and it must be asked how many of the improved outcomes relate to this fact alone. Many doctors would argue that they too would achieve higher patient satisfaction rates with longer consultations, and that this is a feature of the length of time rather than of the skills of the practitioner. This is, of course, entirely possible. Interestingly, Revley (1998) observed that Nurse Practitioners (NPs) made less referrals to the Practice Nurse (PN) than did GPs (5.6% for the NPs, 29% for the GPs). Although the reasons for these referrals is not explored, it would seem likely that they were for investigations (e.g. blood tests) or treatments (e.g. dressings) which the NP may have done herself in the slightly longer consultation time allotted. The Centre for Innovation in Primary Care (2000) also observed that the time spent with patients was similar for PNs and GPs, but that nurses spent the extra time between consultations in completing the necessary administration that GPs would tend to do during the consultation. They suggest that this might lead to nurses giving the patient their more complete attention during the consultation, and hence to some of the better patient satisfaction outcomes.

One small study set in secondary care examined nurse-led follow-up of lung cancer patients, and traditional medical follow-up (Moore *et al.*, 2002). Again, whilst both groups were satisfied with the care they received, those followed up by nurses were more satisfied and scored significantly higher in each subset measured. However, the model of follow-up adopted by the nurses was entirely different to that followed by the medical staff, and resulted in far more time spent in contact with the patient, either by phone or face to face. It was a very supportive model of follow-up, addressing a wider, more holistic agenda than conventional medical follow-up. This would suggest that it may not only be the extra time spent in nurse consultations that is of value to the patient, it is how the nurse uses that the time and the model of care followed.

Diagnosis

Traditionally, diagnosis has been seen as the prerogative of the medical practitioner, with nurse involvement being informal and often unacknowledged (Baird, 2001; Walby and Greenwall, 1994). However, the Review of Prescribing, Supply and Administration of Medicines [Crown II] (Department of Health, DoH, 1999) stated that part of the role of the independent prescriber is to establish a diagnosis and/or management plan. This would suggest that nurse involvement in diagnosis is now formally acknowledged. Within the context of supplementary prescribing, it is expected that the independent prescriber would be responsible for the initial diagnosis and management plan (see Chapter 1). However, nurses working as supplementary prescribers would be experts within their fields of practice, and would be expected to raise their concerns with the independent prescriber if they suspected an incorrect diagnosis.

It has been suggested (Baird, 2000a, b) that nurses have for a long time been involved in the diagnosis of both acute and chronic disease, with many doctors openly acknowledging and accepting this. However, nurses are wise to remember that their initial training does not equip them for such a role. Many courses of varying quality are being developed to meet this need, but those nurses training as extended/supplementary prescribers should remember that the prescribing course is not in itself designed to teach the clinical skills necessary for diagnosis. Nurses training to prescribe are assumed to already have the necessary clinical skills in the area(s) in which they intend to prescribe.

In reaching a working diagnosis, the practitioner will go through several stages of data collection and analysis. Bates (1995) discusses in some depth the process of clinical decision-making and establishing a working diagnosis, whilst acknowledging that it is not always possible to reach a definite diagnosis. Tate (2003) suggests that particularly within primary care, it may well not always be possible or even desirable to make a firm clinical diagnosis in order to formulate a management plan. For example, the patient presenting with a sore throat may have an illness that is viral or bacterial in origin, but as the management and outcome are essentially the same, there is no real need to differentiate in the majority of cases.

In reality, there will often exist an element of uncertainty about a diagnosis. It has been suggested that nurses can find tolerating uncertainty difficult (Luker, 1998). Traditionally, nurse training has not prepared nurses for this, as the risk has been born by the doctor who has decided on, and taken responsibility for, the treatment. Medical training, in contrast, prepares doctors to make decisions in the face of uncertainty (Fox, 1979; Royal College of General Practitioners (RCGP), 1996). This is something that prescribing nurses will need to learn to manage as they accept responsibility for their own prescribing decisions.

CONSULTATIONS WITH PHARMACISTS

The concept of a pharmacist undertaking a consultation with a patient is also relatively new, though many community pharmacists have been consulting with the public for many years, albeit in an informal and unrecognised manner. Lack of privacy and the need for a private consulting room have been identified as a potential barrier to community pharmacists offering more formal consultations (Bellingham, 2002a). However, a number of pharmacies are already participating in pilot schemes that enable them to supply directly simple remedies to patients who do not pay for their prescriptions (Bellingham, 2002b) and these schemes are likely to be expanded in the future.

Literature on pharmacists consultation skills is sparse, but the recent interest in clinical medication review (DoH, 2001) has led to an increase in the number of practice based pharmacists consulting directly with patients about their medication. Petty et al. (2003) suggest that while such a role is acceptable to a large number of patients, some remain suspicious, and further research is needed into the views of patients and carers. Chen and Britten (2000), in their study of medication reviews, observed that pharmacists conducting such reviews did not seem to experience any significant difficulties in communicating with patients. Consultations were relatively long as compared with nurse or doctor consultations (15–90 minutes) and patients would seem to value being able to spend time with a pharmacist in an unhurried environment. Whilst the style and process of consultation are not explored, patients in this study divulged many of their beliefs about their medication to the pharmacist, many of which they had not felt able to discuss with the prescribing doctor. Whether this is a feature of consulting with a different practitioner to the original prescriber, or is something which pharmacist prescribers would also be able to elicit, is unknown.

Many pharmacists have developed skills in concordance that they will be able to bring to their consultations. Concordance, suggest Weiss and Britten (2003), refers to a consultation process and sharing of power between the professional and the patient. It values the patient's experience of illness and medication as much as the professional's expert knowledge. It is possible that pharmacist prescribers who have already developed expertise in this area may achieve better outcomes in their prescribing practice.

DECISION-MAKING AND PRESCRIBING

Within the context of the consultation, the prescriber will be faced with a number of decisions, including the formulation of a diagnosis or management plan, and whether or not to prescribe (Luker *et al.*, 1998). The nursing and medical literature describes two broad models of decision-making: the *analytical* and the *intuitive*. The analytical model describes a logical process of decision-making (Pauker and Karriser, 1987; Miers, 1990; Harbison, 1991) often using a decision tree or algorithm. A limitation of this method is that it assumes that all relevant knowledge is available to the practitioner, something that is often not the case in practice.

The intuitive model has been extensively discussed by Benner (1984), who describes five stages from novice to expert practitioner. Benner (1984) suggests that the method of decision-making depends upon which stage the nurse is at in her professional development. The novice relies very much on an analytical method of decision-making, as she has no experience to guide her thinking, whilst the expert practitioner also draws on intuitive knowledge gained by experience. Hamm (1988), however, views the analytic and the intuitive models as ends of a continuum, and suggests that practitioners will tend more towards the analytic end of the continuum the more time and information are available. In reality, most clinical decision-making is likely to involve both an analytic and intuitive aspect.

INFLUENCES ON PRESCRIBING

In deciding whether, or what, to prescribe, clinicians are likely to be influenced by a number of factors. It has been suggested (Denig and Bradley, 1998) that these fall into three main categories; pressure from patients; pressure from other prescribers; and other influences. In many cases, it may well be that a prescription is not the most appropriate response, especially in primary care where symptoms may be attributable to 'illness' rather than 'disease' (Stewart and Roter, 1989).

A number of studies have suggested that doctors frequently prescribe in response to pressure from patients, either real or perceived. (Bradley, 1992; Britten, 1994; Vrji and Britten, 1991; Stevenson *et al.*, 1999). It may be that some patients do expect to leave the consultation with a prescription, but this is by no means always the case, and the desire for explanation and reassurance is often underestimated (Britten *et al.*, 2000; Barry *et al.*, 2000). Doctors prescribe in response to patients health beliefs, to preserve the doctor–patient relationship and to end a difficult or lengthy consultation. Non-medical prescribers would be naïve to think that they will be immune from such pressures.

Pressure from other prescribers can also be a factor in deciding on a prescription. Precedents set by 'specialists', prescribing colleagues and possibly even oneself in a previous encounter with the patient, may all influence the outcome of a consultation. The pharmaceutical industry will have new prescribers in its sights, and clinicians are likely to be influenced by all these sources. Trust policies on prescribing will seek to influence prescribers and there may, on occasions, be conflicts between these policies and what the practitioner believes to be in the best interest of the patient. External influences include local formularies, clinical guidelines, National Institute for Clinical Excellence (NICE) guidelines and the National Service Framework (NSFs), and the media, which is increasingly seeking to influence patients more directly. Prescribers will have to negotiate a path through these varying influences.

Hall *et al.* (2003) observed that a number of factors influence community nurses decisions to prescribe, with the need to promote patient concordance emerging as a key influence. Another factor, which may be more pertinent to nurse, rather than GP prescribers, would appear to be whether or not the patient is exempt from prescription charges. Many of the items available to nurse prescribers can be bought, and some (though by no means all) nurses reported being heavily influenced by the patient's status in respect of prescription charges (Luker *et al.*, 1998; Hall, 2000).

PRINCIPLES OF GOOD PRESCRIBING

The National Prescribing Centre (NPC, 1999) has developed a series of 'signposts', known as the 'prescribing pyramid' (Figure 3.1) to assist nurses in decision-making; these would be equally of value to pharmacist prescribers. These seven principles break down the complex process of prescribing into a series of steps, which, if considered, may help practitioners to prescribe appropriately.

- *Consider the patient*: Thorough consideration of the holistic needs of the patient, including medical and social history, can help in deciding whether or not medication is indicated. A drug history, including over the counter (OTC) and alternative therapies should be included, along with any drug allergies or sensitivities.

- *Which strategy?* Treatment options other than prescribing should always be considered, including explanation, reassurance and recommending the buying of OTC medication. The practitioner needs to discover and acknowledge the patient's expectations (Pendleton, 9).

- *Consider the choice of product*: The NPC suggest the use of the mnemonic '*EASE*' to assist in deciding which product to prescribe, i.e.:
    - E – how **E**ffective is the product?
    - A – is it **A**ppropriate for this patient?
    - S – how **S**afe is it?
    - E – is the prescription cost-**E**ffective?

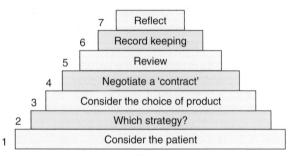

Figure 3.1 The prescribing pyramid NPC (1999). (http://www.npc.co.uk/
nurse_prescribing/bulletins/signposts1.2.htm)

- *Negotiate a contract*: Prescribing should be viewed as shared decision-making between the patient and the prescriber. Effective communication on the part of the prescriber is essential to ensure that the patient understands what the prescription is for, how long it takes to work, how to take it and how long for, what dose to take and any possible side-effects.

- *Reviewing the patient*: It is not good practice to issue repeat prescriptions without regular patient review, and the implementation guidelines for Extended Formulary Nurse Prescribers (DoH, 2002) suggest that nurses should not issue repeat prescriptions for more than six months without reassessment. However, this may lead to some tensions. For example, within general practice, many patients who are well established on the contraceptive pill are only reviewed annually. It would not be reasonable for the practice to have a different approach to those patients who initially saw the nurse. How this will work in practice remains to be seen. In reality, it is likely that those repeat prescriptions which were initiated by other prescribers will be generated by receptionists along with prescriptions initiated by GP, and will be signed by the GP. However, clinicians have a responsibility that goes beyond the initial prescribing decision, and should ensure that they are involved in practice discussions on repeat prescribing policy and medicines management.

- *Keeping records*: The NMC guidelines on record keeping outline the standards expected of all nurses, and there are additional requirements for nurse prescribers to record their prescription in the GP records within 48 hours. Similar standards are expected of pharmacist prescribers (DoH, 2002). Local policy as to how this is to be achieved will vary.

- *Reflect*: Reflecting on prescribing decisions, both alone or with colleagues, (possibly within the context of clinical supervision), will help practitioners to improve and develop their prescribing practice.

COMPUTER DECISION SUPPORT

With the proliferation of information technology in healthcare, the interest in computerised support has increased. A number of systems to assist in the process of decision-making and prescribing have been developed, including Prodigy (www.prodigy.nhs.uk), which is well known in general practice; Isabel, (www.isabel.org.uk) a tool to support differential diagnosis in paediatric practice; and the Clinical Assessment System (CAS) used by NHS direct. Given the ever increasing scope of medical knowledge, and the vast number of potential treatments, there is no doubt that these systems should be able to facilitate better decision making, though how best to integrate them in the consultation remains a challenge (Eccles *et al.*, 2002). There is a suggestion that those systems which interrupt the consultation with prompts are less well received by practitioners that those which can be accessed 'on demand' (Rousseau *et al.*, 2003). It has also been suggested (Sullivan, 1995) that using a computer within the consultation can tend to increase the doctor-initiated, 'medical' content of the consultation, at the expense of patient-initiated and 'social' content, whilst increasing the length of the consultation. However, there is no doubt that computers are here to stay, and used appropriately, they may have the potential to improve clinician performance (Sullivan, 1995).

CONCLUSION

Nurses and pharmacists have sought the ability to prescribe for many years. It brings with it a new level of responsibility and accountability, and has the potential to alter the dynamics of the practitioner/patient relationship. Skills in communication and decision making are central to this relationship, whether or not the practitioner is a prescriber. Those new to prescribing may need to ensure that the ability to issue a prescription does not detract from other, equally important aspects of their relationship with the patient.

References

Baird A (2000a). Crown II: The implications of Nurse Prescribing for Practice Nurses. *British Journal of Community Nursing* **5(9)**: 454–461.

Baird A (2000b). Prescribing decisions in general practice. *Practice Nursing* **11(7)**: 9–12.

Baird A (2001). Diagnosis and prescribing. *Primary Healthcare* **11(5)**: 24–26.

Bates B (1995). *A Guide to Physical Examination and History Taking* 6th edn. Philadelphia: JB Lippincott Company.

Barry CA, Bradley CP, Britten N *et al.* (2000). Patients unvoiced agendas in general practice consultations. *British Medical Journal* **320**: 1246–1250.

Bellingham C (2002a). Space, time and team working: issues for pharmacists who wish to prescribe. *The Pharmaceutical Journal* **268**: 562–563.

Bellingham C (2002). Pharmacists who prescribe: the reality. *The Pharmaceutical Journal* **268**: 238–239.

Benner P (1984). From novice to expert. *Excellence and Power in Clinical Nursing Practice*. California: Addison Wesley Publishing Company.

Bond S, Beck S, Cunningham F *et al.* (1999). Testing a rating scale of video-taped consultations to assess performance of trainee nurse practitioners in General Practice. *Journal of Advanced Nursing* **30(5)**.

Bradley CP (1992). Uncomfortable prescribing decisions: a critical incident study. *British Medical Journal* **304**: 294–296.

Britten N (1994). Patient Demand for Prescriptions. A view from the other side. *Family Practice* **11**: 62–66.

Britten N, Stevenson F, Barry A *et al.* (2000). Misunderstandings in prescribing decisions in general practice: a qualitative study. *British Medical Journal* **320**: 484–488.

Byrne PS, Long BEL (1976). *Doctors Talking to Patients.* London: HMSO.

Chant S, Jenkinson T, Randle J *et al.* (2002). Communication skills: some problems in nurse education and practice. *Journal of Clinical Nursing* **11(1)**: 12–21.

Chen J, Britten N (2000). 'String Medicine': an analysis of pharmacist consultations in primary care. *Family Practice* **17(6)**: 480–483.

Department of Health (1999). *Review of Prescribing Supply and Administration of Medicines (Crown Copyright).* London: DoH.

Department of Health (2001). *Medicines and Older People: implementing medicines related aspects of the National Service Framework for Older People.* London: DoH.

Department of Health (2002). *Extending Independent Nurse Prescribing within the NHS in England (Crown Copyright).* London: DoH.

Denig P, Bradley C (1998). How doctors choose drugs In*: Prescribing in Primary Care* (Hobbs R and Bradley C). Oxford: Oxford Medical Publications.

Drucquer M, Hutchinson S (2000). *The Consultation Toolkit. A Practical Method for Teaching and Learning Consultation Skills.* Surrey: Reed Healthcare Publishing.

Eccles M, McColl E, Steen N *et al.* (2002). Effect of computerised evidence based guidelines on management of asthma and angina in adults in primary care: cluster randomised controlled trial. *British Medical Journal* **325**: 941–947.

Fox R (1979). *Essays in Medical Sociology.* New York: John Wiley and Sons.

Greco M, Powell R (2003). A Patient feedback tool. *Primary Healthcare* **12(10)**: 38–41.

Hall J, Cantrill J, Noyce P (2003). Influences on community nurse prescribing. *Nurse Prescribing* **1(3)**: 127–132.

Harbison J (1991). Clinical decision making in nursing. *Journal of Advanced Nursing* **16**: 404–407.

Hamm RM (1988). Clinical intuition and clinical analysis: expertise and the cognitive continuum. In: *Professional Judgement – a reader in clinical decision making* (Dowie, J and Elstein, A). Cambridge: Cambridge University Press.

Horrocks S, Anderson E, Salisbury C (2002). Systematic review of whether nurse practitioners working in primary care can provide equivalent care to doctors. *British Medical Journal* **324**: 819–823.

Kemm J, Close A (1995). *Health Promotion Theory and Practice.* London: Macmillan Press Ltd.

Kinnersley P, Anderson E, Parry K *et al.* (2000). Randomised controlled trial of nurse practitioner versus general practitioner care for patients requesting 'same day' consultations in primary care. *British Medical Journal* **320**: 1043.

Launer J (2002). Narrative based primary care. *A Practical Guide.* Oxon: Radcliffe Medical Press.

Luker K, Hogg C, Austin L *et al.* (1998). Decision making: the context of nurse prescribing. *Journal of Advanced Nursing* **27**: 657–665.

Maguire P, Pitceathy C (2002). Key communication skills and how to acquire them *British Medical Journal* **325**: 697–700.

Miers M (1990). Developing skills in decision making. *Nursing Times* **86(30)**: 32–33.

Moore S, Corner J, Haviland J *et al.* (2002). Nurse led follow up and conventional medical follow up in management of patients with lung cancer: randomised trial. *British Medical Journal* **325**: 1145–1147.

National Prescribing Centre (1999). Signposts for prescribing nurses – general principles of good prescribing. *Nurse Prescribing Bulletin.* **1(1)**. (http://www.npc.co.uk/nurse_prescribing/bulletins/signposts1.1.htm).

Neighbour R (1987). *The Inner Consultation: How to Develop an Effective and Intuitive Consulting Style.* Lancaster: MTP Press.

Pendleton D, Schofield T, Tate P *et al.* (1984). *The Consultation: An Approach to Learning and Teaching.* Oxford: Oxford University Press.

Pauker SG, Karriser JP (1987). Medical progress decision analysis. *New England Journal of Medicine* **316(5)**: 250–258.

Petty DR, Knapp P, Raynor DK, House AO (2003). Patients' views of a pharmacist-run medication review clinic in general practice. *British Journal of General Practice* **53**: 607–613.

Revley S (1998). The role of the triage nurse practitioner in general medical practice: an analysis of the role. *Journal of Advanced Nursing* **28(3)**: 584–591.

Rotter JB (1954). *Social Learning and Clinical Psychology.* Englewood Cliffs, NJ: Prentice-Hall.

Rosenstock IM (1974). The health belief model and preventative health behaviour. In: *The Health Belief Model and Personal Health Behaviour* (Becker, M). Thorafore, NJ: Charles Slack.

Rousseau N, McColl E, Newton J *et al.* Practice based, longitudinal, qualitative interview study of computerised evidence based guidelines in primary care. *British Medical Journal* **326**: 314–322.

Royal College of General Practitioners (1996). *The Nature of General Medical Practice.* London: RCGP.

Shum C, Humphreys A, Wheeler D *et al.* (2000). Nurse management of patients with minor illness in general practice: multicentre, randomised controlled trial. *British Medical Journal* **320**: 1038–1043.

Silverman J, Kurtz S, Draper J (1998). *Skills for Communicating with Patients.* Radcliffe Oxon: Medical Press.

Stewart MA, Roter D (1989) Eds. *Communicating with Medical Patients.* Newbury Park: Sage Publications.

Sullivan F and Mitchell E (1995). Has general practitioner computing made a difference to patient care? A systematic review of published reports. *British Medical Journal* **311**: 848–852.

Tate (2003). *The Doctor's Communication Handbook* 4th edn. Oxon: Radcliffe Medical Press.

The Centre for Innovation in Primary Care (2000). *What Do Practice Nurses Do? A Study of Roles, Responsibilities and Patterns of Work.* The Centre for Innovation in Primary Care, Sheffield (www.innovate.org.uk).

Stott NCH and Davies RH (1979). The exceptional potential in each primary care consultation. *Journal of the Royal College of General Practitioners* **29**: 210–215.

Virji A, Britten N (1991). A study of the relationship between patients' attitudes and doctors' prescribing. *Family Practice* **8**: 314–319.

Walby S, Greenwall J (1994). *Medicine and Nursing: Professions in a Changing Health Service.* London: Sage.

Weiss M, Britten N (2003). What is concordance? *The Pharmaceutical Journal* **271**: 493.

While A (2002). Practical skills: prescribing consultation in practice. *British Journal of Community Nursing* **7(9)**: 469–473.

Chapter 4

Legal aspects of independent and supplementary prescribing

Mark Gagan

It seems that legal issues are a constant source of worry and fascination for many healthcare practitioners. Litigation costs have soared through the 1990s and one estimate has put the costs in the region of £4 billion (Tingle, 2002).

Since 1997, there have been many reviews, revisions and changes to the way the National Health Services (NHS) provides care. Most of these changes are due to Governmental policy, some are because of the response to systemic failures such as the Bristol Royal Infirmary affair (http://www.dh.gov.uk/PublicationsAnd Statistics/Publications/PublicationsPolicyAndGuidance/PublicationsPolicyAndGui-danceArticle/fs/en?CONTENT_ID=4009387&chk=LnDPof) and the Alder Hey Organ retention scandal in Liverpool (http://www.dh.gov.uk/PublicationsAnd-Statistics/Publications/PublicationsPolicyAndGuidance/PublicationsPolicyAndGui-danceArticle/fs/en?CONTENT_ID=4005937&chk=st0wM3) Others are because of the increasing expectations of the general public who are arguably better informed of their rights than ever before.

This chapter sets out to give a précise of the history of changes brought about by the desire to change prescribing authority, give definitions of independent and supplementary prescribing, patient group directions (PGD) and their possible implications for practitioners.

There is a short introduction to how the law is formulated, the differences between civil and criminal law and how issues such as duty of care, negligence, consent and accountability might affect interactions with patients. Professional issues such as teamwork and communication are also addressed. Cases that have gone before the courts are highlighted in an attempt to illustrate how the law has been previously applied. The role of professional bodies is also considered in some detail throughout.

LEGISLATION RELEVANT TO PRESCRIBING INCLUDES

The Medicines Act, 1968 regulates the licensing, supply and administration of medicines.

The act also requires the Secretary of State for Health to place on the prescription only list, medicines that represent a danger to patients if their use is not super-vised by an appropriate practitioner. (Medicines Act 1968, s58(2)(b) cited in Griffith *et al.*, 2003.)

It also classifies medicines into three categories:

Prescription-only-medicines

These are medicines, which may be supplied or administered on the instruction of an appropriate practitioner (a doctor or dentist) and from an approved list for a nurse prescriber. The pharmacist is the expert on all aspects of medicines legislation and should be consulted.

Pharmacy-only-medicines

These can be purchased from a registered primary care pharmacy, provided the pharmacist supervises the sale.

General sales list

These need neither a prescription nor the supervision of a pharmacist and can be obtained from retail outlets.

The act also states the following points:

- An appropriate practitioner is: 'a doctor, dentist or veterinary surgeon'.

- A specific prescription is always required for the supply of a prescription-only-medicines (POMs).

- A prescription for POMs has to come from 'an appropriate practitioner'.

- A POM can be administered by a doctor, dentist or veterinary surgeon or a 'person acting on the instruction of an appropriate practitioner' only (Pennells, 1999).

This means that only those who are stated to be 'appropriate practitioners' can prescribe POMs. Obviously, this does not include nurses, midwives or other allied health professionals.

The Cumberledge Report, 1986 was the first suggestion that community nurses should have prescribing rights (Tingle, 1998).

The First Crown Report, 1989 recommended that health visitors and community nurses should have the power to prescribe medication from a 'nurses' formulary' in order to benefit patients.

The Medicinal Product: Prescribing for Nurses Act, 1992 further opened the process of prescribing by stating that those nurses on parts 1 and 12 (Registered General Nurses, RGNs) of the UKCC register who also possessed a district nursing qualification or who were on part 11 of the register (health visitors) or on part 10 of the register (midwives) and who had undergone further training, had a legal right to prescribe products from a very limited list (Pennells, 1999). This list was known as the Nurse Prescriber's Formulary (NPF).

The success of nurse prescribing encouraged legislators to further the cause. The *Pharmaceutical Services Regulations, 1994* were changed to allow pharmacists to legally accept and dispense prescriptions written by nurses (Gibson, 2001). *The second Crown Report 1999 (Review of prescribing, supply and administrations of Medicines)* proposed the introduction of a new framework of prescribing, supply and administrations of medicines whereby the majority of patients would receive medicines on an individual patient-specific basis, the prescribing authority of doctors, dentists, district nurses and health visitors would continue and that this prescribing authority would be extended to include new groups of healthcare professionals (Department of Health, DoH, 2003).

Nurses would be expected to complete a rigorous training course, taught to a level 3 (degree) standard by an approved Higher Education Institute (HEI) and be supervised in practice by an appropriate clinician (see Nursing and Midwifery Council (NMC) Circular 25/2002).

Pharmacists also would be expected to follow broadly the same type of curriculum specifically appropriate to their needs.

The practice competencies necessary for prescribing have been considered by the National Prescribing Centre (NPC) and outline frameworks for both nurses and pharmacists have been established (NPC, 2003).

DEFINITIONS OF 'INDEPENDENT' AND 'SUPPLEMENTARY' PRESCRIBER

Independent prescribing 'means that the prescriber takes responsibility for the clinical assessment of the patient, establishing a diagnosis and the clinical management required, as well as for prescribing where necessary and the appropriateness of any prescription'.

DoH (2003)

There are two types of independent prescriber, IP (other than doctors, dentists or veterinary surgeons)

- Those district nurses and health visitors who, following training, are permitted to prescribe from the NPF.
- The 'Extended Formulary Nurse Prescriber', a first level Registered Nurse or Registered Midwife, who after following a specific training programme, will be able to prescribe from the Nurse Prescribers' Extended Formulary (DoH, 2003). These medicines to be prescribed in the areas of minor illness, minor injury, health promotion and palliative care.

Supplementary Prescribing is defined as 'a voluntary partnership between an IP (a doctor or a dentist) and a supplementary prescriber (SP; a nurse or pharmacist) to implement an agreed patient-specific Clinical Management Plan (CMP) with the patients agreement'.

DoH (2003)

There will be no legal restrictions placed on the clinical conditions that may be treated under supplementary prescribing, although there is an expectation that supplementary prescribing would be used for chronic medical conditions and health needs.

PGD is defined as 'a written instruction for the supply or administration of medicines to groups of patients who may not be individually identified before presentation for treatment. It is not a form of prescribing and there is no specific training that health professionals must undertake before supplying or administering medicines in this way' (DoH, 2003). Further guidance is available in Health Service Circular 2000/26.

This changed form of prescribing authority commenced in England (for nurse pre-scribers at least) from April 2003. The other countries of the UK will need to look to their own devolved governments for information on planned strategies and the timetable for their implementation.

It is important to have an awareness of these definitions, as the practitioner may be called upon in a court of law (or to answer before their own professional body or employing authority) to defend their practice against accusations of malprac-tice. There are several important examples of healthcare professionals having to face such allegations and these will be used to illustrate the importance of under-standing the legal process.

THE LEGAL SYSTEM IN ENGLAND

In essence there are two branches of law; civil and criminal.

Civil law usually deals with disputes where one person who has suffered loss or harm (the plaintiff) brings a legal action against another person (known as the defendant) who the plaintiff believes has caused them the loss or the harm (Tingle, 1998). This might be referred to as a 'tort' or a civil wrong; these might include negligence, or assault (due to lack of valid consent). If these torts are proven, the plaintiff can claim damages (usually financial recompense) against the defendant (Tingle, 1998). Criminal law is mostly concerned with offences against the state (the law of the land rather than private individuals) and it is usually the Crown that brings the action against the defendant.

There is also a system of courts, both civil and criminal, that deal with all actions in law.

In civil courts, the actions are usually presented before a judge who makes a deci-sion on the evidence presented before the court. In criminal cases, most actions start at the local magistrates' court and then move on, depending upon the sever-ity of the alleged offence. In serious cases, the evidence may be presented to a judge and jury. In these cases, it is the jury who decide whether the defendant is guilty, or not guilty, of the alleged offence.

SOURCES OF LAW

The law of the land is primarily made using two devices.

Statutes

Statutes are Acts of Parliament, which are presented via the House of Commons following an established process that involves debate and argument before being moved on to the House of Lords. Here, there is further debate and requests for changes (amendments) are usually made before the statutes are returned to the House of Commons. On completion of the debates, the 'bill' is given royal assent (the approval of the reigning monarch) and passes into law.

Common law (sometimes known as judge-made law)

In cases where there is no existing Act of Parliament to cover a particular occurrence, the legal system looks for similar cases that have been decided in the past by judges.

There is a legal term known as 'precedent', which indicates that cases showing similar facts and similar progressions to previous cases should be dealt with in a 'like-for-like manner'. This system works on the premise that the higher the court is in the legal system, the more binding its decisions are on the courts below them. The highest court in England is that of the House of Lords and its decisions are followed by every other court in the land (although there is now the possibility that certain cases can go before the European Court, as the UK is a member of the European Union, and subject, in certain circumstances, to European law). The fact that judges act in a certain manner because of precedent has important implications for prescribers, particularly in cases where negligence or duty of care standards are being considered.

NEGLIGENCE

Montgomery (2002) suggests that to win a negligence case it is necessary (for the plaintiff) to prove three things:

1. At the time of mishap, the defendant had responsibility for the care of the plaintiff (i.e. they had a 'duty of care').

2. That the standard of care given did not reach that required by law (essentially, a level acceptable to the defendant's professional peers).

3. That the failure to act properly, and not some other factor, caused the injuries received.

If any of these three factors is untenable, the case will fail. If all are present, then the burden of proof rests on 'the balance of probabilities' (i.e. a reasonable degree of probability that the tort was caused by the defendant). The standard of civil proof is less than that for criminal cases where it must be established beyond reasonable doubt that the person is guilty of a particular act.

DUTY OF CARE

The plaintiff has to prove that the healthcare professional owed a duty of care to him/her.

The legal precedent for establishing duty of care can be exemplified in *Donaghue versus Stevenson [1932] AC 562* where a manufacturer was held liable for the injuries received by the plaintiff who consumed a bottle of ginger beer that contained the remains of a decomposed snail and as a result developed gastro-enteritis. This case produced the 'neighbour principle' which states that a duty of care is owed to anyone who is reasonably likely to be affected by one's acts or omissions (Hendrick, 2000). It can be argued that patients are likely to come into the category of 'neighbour' (Gibson, 2001). Although it might appear highly unlikely that a bottle of ginger beer and snail remains can have an adverse effect on a practitioner's status, it must be remembered that when 'precedent' is applied, the circumstances of one case can be applied to another, even if it appears to have little in common at first glance.

Once duty of care has been established, it has to be shown that the practitioner failed to honour that commitment and caused a breach of that duty to occur. The practitioner's actions would have to be examined to see if they reached an accepted level of competence.

The legal standard of care is classically defined in the case of *Bolam versus Friern Hospital Management Committee [1957] 1 WLR 582* cited by Montgomery (2002) where it was stated that 'a doctor is not held guilty of negligence, if he has acted in accordance with a practice accepted as proper by a responsible body of medical men skilled in that particular art'. The language may seem archaic now, but the application of the principle is crucial. It need not be 'medical men' that are being judged; it could be nurses, pharmacists, midwives or community practitioners. The names are not that important – it is the job being done that is under scrutiny.

This is an important benchmark for practitioners as it implies that they will be judged against the standards of their peers, by their peers. The courts might set the test but it is up to these professionals to decide whether or not the test has been passed. This may seem to favour the professional rather than the plaintiff and this has been a source of debate for many years. This situation is at present being questioned by senior judges, who appear to indicate that a degree of scepticism may be useful when considering the evidence of expert peers.

The notion that 'doctor knows best' is no longer considered a cast iron guarantee of certainty, particularly following the *Bolitho* case. This case involved the treatment of a young child, who it was claimed suffered injury through the neglect of a doctor who refused to come to see him when requested. The child's condition was very serious and it was unlikely that he would have survived, even if the doctor concerned had intubated him. An expert at the time of the trial supported this case. This rationale did not win the support of the Law Lords, who felt that risks should be weighed up and balanced, so that practice could be logically and rigorously defended (see later discussion).

The final stage in the process of proving negligence is to examine if any damage or injury occurred as a result of the practitioner's actions. If it can be shown that the action taken by the practitioner was inappropriate and that it could reasonably be foreseen that damage or injury would occur as a result of the practitioner's actions, then it could be stated that the charge of negligence is well founded. The practitioner would be liable for damages (fiscal compensation, and possibly costs from both parties if these are awarded by the court against the practitioner) and may face disciplinary action by their employer.

The legal situation may be less problematic for the practitioner than the professional body's view of the standard of competence demonstrated by their registered members.

The practitioner may not have broken any criminal laws, despite their care being deemed less than what would normally be expected. However, the professional body might feel that, by his or her actions, the practitioner has brought the profession into disrepute. If the professional body, after hearing evidence from all concerned parties, decides that the actions taken were unacceptable, then the practitioner may face punishment ranging from cautions about future conduct to removal from the professional register. The latter sanction can have dire effects on the practitioner's ability to remain employed, as removal from professional registers means that a person is no longer entitled to call themselves (at least in the case of Nurses) a Registered Nurse.

TEAMWORK

In supplementary prescribing, the interaction between the IP (a doctor or dentist) and the SP is maintained on a voluntary basis.

The working relationship is expected to be a close one between the professionals and it should be noted 'good prescribing practice requires that the patient is considered an equal partner in order to ensure informed consent and concordance'. (The Task Force on Medicines Partnership, 2002 cited NPC, 2003). Most legal authorities would encourage this openness and sharing, as it indicates a willingness to engage patients in a transparent manner (see Consent).

RESPONSIBILITIES OF PRESCRIBING PARTNERS

Prescribing partners must work together in an open, co-operative manner that ensures lawful supplementary prescribing is upheld. This means that:

- The IP is a doctor, dentist or registered nurse prescriber.
- The SP is a registered nurse, registered midwife or registered pharmacist.
- A written care plan exists relating to a named patient and to that patient's specific conditions. Agreement to the plan must be recorded by both the independent and SP before supplementary prescribing begins.
- The independent and SP share, have access to, consult, and use the same patient record.

NPC (2003)

These aspirations are echoed in the NMC Code of Conduct (NMC, 2002) particularly in Clause 8.1 which stipulates:

'You must work with other members of the team to promote healthcare environments that are conducive to safe, therapeutic and ethical practice. Though not all independent and SPs are nurses, the exhortation is one aspiring to best practice, which is something all prescribers should be working towards'.

If a situation arose where a case of negligence was brought that involved a SP, a defence of 'team' rather than 'individual' responsibility for the error, would not be a valid defence. In law, there is no such thing as 'team liability'. This was shown in the case of *Prendergast versus Sam Dee [1989 Med LR 36]* where a doctor prescribed amoxil but the writing was so illegible that the pharmacist thought daonil had been prescribed and dispensed this to the patient instead. Unfortunately, the patient became permanently brain damaged as a result of the error. The court found in favour of the plaintiff and awarded damages of over £139,000. The doctor was found to be 25% liable, with the remaining sum awarded against the pharmacist. Best practice would suggest that each practitioner is personally and professionally accountable for their own actions performed in the course of their work.

Clause 1.3 of the NMC Code of professional conduct states:

You are personally accountable for your practice. This means you are answerable for your actions and omissions, regardless of advice or directions from another professional.

NMC (2002)

This underlines the importance of being able to defend decisions made in the course of practice. Research-based care delivered promptly and appropriately is becoming the 'gold standard' approach to interactions with patients. This is highlighted in the case of *Bolitho versus City and Hackney Health Authority [1997] 4 All ER 771 HL* in which a young child suffered brain damage following a cardiac arrest. One of the main issues in the case was whether the doctor's failure to intubate a child (who had previously the same afternoon suffered two apparent airway occlusions) contributed to the cardiac arrest. If the doctor did not intubate the child, would this be unreasonable behaviour and the doctor would fall short of their duty of care to the child. It was found that there was a reasonable body of expert opinion to suggest that it might be considered reasonable not to intubate the child and thus, the doctor was not liable under the Bolam test.

Since the *Bolitho* case, it has become accepted that judges look to more than expert opinion when deciding on the merits of particular practices performed by practitioners.

Not only must the practitioner perform their duties to a specific standard (as suggested by the Bolam test) but that standard must also be able to be defended logically and supported by credible evidence. Lord Woolfe, the Lord Chief Justice in 2001, stated that the phrase 'doctor knows best' (perhaps with the Bolam test in mind) might be better phrased, 'doctor knows best if he acts reasonably and logically and gets his facts right' (cited in Tingle, 2002).

It is a real challenge to the notion that the experts know best and that this is sufficient reason to believe what they say. It is a call to practitioners to be fully accountable and in doing so, be able to defend their care from a sound basis.

This is supported by the NMC Code of professional conduct, (2002), Clause 6.1, which states:

> You must keep your knowledge and skills up to date throughout your working life. In particular, you should take part regularly in learning activities that develop your competence and performance and in Clause 6.5:

> You have a responsibility to deliver care based on current evidence, best practice and, where applicable, validated research when it is available.

This has implications for lifelong learning and the application of evidence-based research into everyday practice. Practitioners' knowledge and competence cannot remain static because the delivery of care is dynamic, with new treatments and techniques being introduced almost on a daily basis. The law requires practitioners to demonstrate an awareness of the new methods of practice. This is exemplified in the case of *Gascoine versus Ian Sheridan and Co and Latham [1994] 5 Med LR 437* cited in Hendrick (2000) where a consultant was questioned on his responsibility to keep up to date with changes in techniques that affected his particular field of expertise. The judge in the case agreed that professionals had a duty to keep informed of mainstream changes but need not be aware of every change that occurred, as this would prove to be time-consuming and difficult to maintain.

In the field of independent and supplementary prescribing, where policy initiatives drive changes forward very quickly and new drugs are being produced at a dramatic rate, it would be impractical to be aware of every development as it happened.

Nonetheless, refreshing one's knowledge and practice regularly will be expected by employers and consumers. This is particularly apposite if a practitioner prescribes a product that, by virtue of its manufacture or because of inappropriate administration or poor instruction, causes damage to the patient.

CONSUMER PROTECTION ACT 1987

This act can be used to bring a claim where a defective product has caused harm.

This is defined as ... *there is a defect in a product ... if the safety of the product is not such that as persons are entitled to expect* ... (Consumer Protection Act 1987 s3(1) cited in Dimond, 2002).

The plaintiff, as such, does not have to prove the defendant negligent, rather that the prescriber had used a defective product. The outcome of this legislation is that a prescriber who gives a medication or dressing to a patient that is found to be defective in some way and causes the patient harm is potentially liable as a supplier of the defective product under the act. The supplier could, therefore, be an independent (doctor, nurse) or SP (pharmacist, nurse). This has implications for understanding the supply mechanisms in the organisation within which one works and using a system where checks can be made that would enable a product to be traced back to its original source (its supplier).

The practitioner, as in all cases, must be knowledgeable about the product supplied and be aware of the potential problems that can arise with its use. Recording of any potential or actual problem would be desirable, along with the circumstances of the occurrence. Careful checking of information on how to use the particular product, its storage, disposal and anticipated effects and the recording of what had been shown to and discussed with the patient with regard to the product would indicate that reasonable care had been taken to inform the patient, should a case come to litigation. The practitioner is also responsible for notifying the appropriate authorities of any adverse drug reactions: Committee on the Safety of Medicines (CSM) and the Medicines Control Agency (MCA) under the 'Yellow Card warning scheme' (see Chapters 2 and 7), a process to help identify any problems with medications at an early stage. This information is collated on a national basis with the aim that close observation and prompt reporting of any untoward events will enhance patient safety.

CONSENT

The expectations of the courts and professional bodies regarding consent are very demanding. There are several important cases that have helped shaped the way courts have dealt with practitioners who have acted without consent. One such case is *Scholendorff versus New York Hospital (1914) 105 NE 92* in which Judge Cardozo established that each adult person, being of sound mind, has the right to accept or refuse medical treatment (including the taking of prescribed medication). To force treatment upon them without their acceptance (or unless allowed to by a court order) is to commit the offence of trespass (even assault or battery) to that person. This can lead to prosecution in a court of law. Although this case is an example of the law of the USA, the similar system of lawmaking adopted that in England means that, occasionally, these judgements are used to inform and support judgements in English Law. The 'Cardozo Judgement' is one such example. All healthcare professional bodies insist that their members seek the consent of the person involved before they engage in any treatment, thereby not opening themselves up to accusations of malpractice. The NMC Code of Conduct (2002) is clear about the responsibilities of nurses and midwives in this respect. Clause 3 (and its accompanying sections) states:

As a registered nurse or midwife, you must obtain consent before you give any treatment or care.

There then follows a series of instructions regarding the validity of consent and how informed consent should be given. This is an important part of the process of consent since, without informed consent, the consent given may well be termed 'invalid' and therefore not recognised in law. Practitioners must ensure that when obtaining consent, it is given by a legally competent person able to understand and retain the information given, thereby making an informed choice about their treatment. This consent must be given voluntarily. The person also has the right to refuse treatment, even if this appears to fly in the face of logic or reason (as far as the practitioner is concerned).

This right was supported in *Re C (an adult) (refusal of medical treatment) Family division 1994 1 All ER 819* (cited in Dimond, 2002). This case concerned a patient incarcerated in a special hospital who had developed gangrene in his leg, which if untreated, would probably kill him. The recommended course of treatment was amputation of the diseased limb. The man refused and took his case to court where it was established that, despite his illness, he had understood the reasons why an operation was deemed necessary and the likely consequences of his refusal to consent to the amputation.

The court found in his favour and declared him legally competent to refuse the operation despite the concerns of the healthcare professionals caring for him. This can be most distressing for the staff but they must respect the autonomy of the patient.

The case highlights the importance of open, honest communication between the practitioner and the patient. It should also encourage practitioners to be dutiful in their assessment of a patient's understanding of procedures or treatments that might be prescribed for them and to carefully record the interaction and information given.

The patient has the right to expect honest, truthful information and the right to request further clarification and a second opinion if they wish.

How much information needs to be given? A simple answer might be along the lines that the amount of information given must be enough to enable the person to reach an informed decision about the pros and cons of following or declining to follow the course of treatment prescribed.

Once this information has been given and considered, and the patient has made their decision to freely give their consent to treatment, the practitioner cannot be accused of acting without consent. The use of concise, factual, contemporaneous written records, indicating what information had been discussed and agreed upon by the patient and practitioner would also be a useful safeguard in case of confusion or if a dispute arose at a later date.

In a famous case: *Sidaway versus Board of Governors of Bethlem Royal Hospital [1985] AC 871; [1985] 1 All ER 1018, HL*, a patient claimed that she had not been given enough warnings about the potential side-effects of an operation she had decided to undergo. The chances of paralysis were reckoned to be very small, but following the procedure, she did suffer from loss of function. The surgeon in charge of the case was accused of negligence, on the grounds that he had not explained the risk of paralysis (however small) to her.

Mrs Sidaway contended that as she had not been made aware of this potential problem, she could not have made an informed choice and her consent was therefore, in effect, invalid.

The case reached the House of Lords, where it was declared that the surgeon who performed the operation had not failed in his duty of care to Mrs Sidaway as he had acted in accordance with a '*practice accepted as proper by a responsible body of neuro-surgical opinion*'. This is a reaffirmation of the criteria applied in the Bolam test, the benchmark of competent practice. The view of the courts, although influenced by judgements such as *Bolitho*, still appears to centre around the Bolam standard, intimating that the information given must meet the competence standard expressed in that case, that of the care accepted as competent by a professional's peers. This would include, in the case of nurses and midwives, any provisions about competent practice in the Code of Professional Conduct (Clauses 1, 2, 3, 6 and 8, in particular).

Professionals also need to remember that no one person can agree to consent to treatment for another adult person. A husband could not consent to treatment to a wife, or a sister to treatment for her sister, for example.

If treatment needed to be performed on an adult person who was incapable (for whatever reason) of giving their informed consent for that treatment, then a doctor might decide to act in the 'best interest' of the patient. The doctor would have to consider the situation extremely carefully and if, in their medical judgement or opinion, the treatment was vital to the patient's well being, they could instigate the treatment, despite the absence of expressed consent, in the best interest of the patient.

It would then be up to the patient to show that the doctor acted in an unlawful manner in subjecting them to that particular treatment in that specific case.

It is not unknown for courts to issue treatment orders against the specific wishes of patients using the rationale of 'best interest'. The case of *Re MB (Adult; Medical treatment) [1997] 2 FLR 426 CA* showed how the courts can view an emergency situation and decide that certain factors (such as pain, fear and drugs) can render a patient 'incompetent' to make an informed decision regarding the acceptance or refusal of medical treatment and in those types of circumstance, they can order treatment to be administered in the 'best interest' of the patient. The case cited related to the delivery of a child by a caesarean operation. The mother had initially consented to the procedure, but withdrew consent on realising that she would have to have an anaesthetic administered by hypodermic injection. The mother had a 'needle phobia' and was adamant that she would not be injected at any time. The court ordered that she should undergo the procedure and that the staff could use means necessary to undertake the operation without the mother's express permission. The child was delivered safely.

This step was not taken lightly by the court, which emphasised the urgent nature of the situation in this case in reaching its decision to override the wishes of the individual.

These situations are problematic for all concerned. Professional bodies indicate what they consider best practice in these circumstances. In the case of nurses and midwives, Clauses 3 and 4 of the Code of Professional Conduct are particularly appropriate in this type of situation.

CONCLUSION

These are dynamic times in the world of independent and supplementary prescribing.

Patients have become much more involved in their treatment and are generally better informed about their rights to healthcare. The need for autonomous, evidence-based practice has never been greater. The law demands that professionals involve patients in all stages of their care, giving them information to make reasonable and appropriate decisions concerning their well being. The need for practitioners who can assess, plan, implement and evaluate the care required and be able to justify that care is increasing. These practitioners must be aware of the need to promote a relationship with the patient that encompasses the physical, emotional, spiritual, ethical and legal implications of this partnership. Professional healthcare bodies encourage their members to be 'knowledgeable doers', displaying all the competencies that this requires. The legal system supplies the 'test' that will show the standard of competence expected – it is up to the healthcare professionals to apply that test and decide if the standard has been reached. One of the defining characteristics of a profession is the autonomy of its members. It is that autonomy that enables us to be called 'professional'. For some practitioners, the freedom this brings can be very satisfying, for they find they can meet a patient's needs much more quickly as a result of this autonomy. In some cases, the freedom to act, instead of releasing the talents (to use another modern phrase) of a practitioner, can inhibit them, by making them wary of the potential problems of falling foul of the law. This is a great pity, as professionals should have a healthy respect for the law and not become so intimidated by it that it hampers, rather than supports, safe practice.

In the final analysis, each practitioner is accountable for his or her practice. If they are unsure of how to perform appropriately, it would be better that they refer to a senior colleague, professional body (or trade union) or Code of Practice, for advice and support. It would be preferable to stop and seek guidance, rather than continue 'blindly' and make a fatal error that would impact badly on the patient and the practitioner themselves.

References

Department of Health (1989). *Report of the Advisory group on Nurse Prescribing (Crown Report).* London: DoH.

Department of Health (1999). *Reveiw of Prescribing, Supply and Administration of Medicines (Crown Report).* London: DoH.

Department of Health (2003). *Supplementary Prescribing by Nurses and Pharmacists within the NHS in England. A Guide for Implementation.* London: DoH.

Department of Health and Social Security (1986). *Neighbourhood Nursing: A focus for Care (Cumberledge Report).* London: DoH.

Dimond B (2002). *Legal Aspects of Nursing* 3rd edn. Harlow: Pearson Education.

Gibson B (2001). Legal and professional accountability for nurse prescribing. In: *Current Issues in Nurses Prescribing* (Courtney, M). London: Greenwich Medical Media Ltd.

Health Care Circular 2002/26. London: DoH.

Hendrick J (2000). *Law and Ethics in Nursing and Health Care.* Cheltenham: Stanley Thornes (Publishers) Ltd.

Montgomery J (2003). *Health Care Law* 2nd edn. Oxford: Oxford University Press.

National Prescribing Centre (2003). *Supplementary Prescribing. A Resource to Help Healthcare Professionals to Understand the Framework and Opportunities.* Liverpool: NPC.

Nursing and Midwifery Council (2002). *Code of Professional Conduct.* London: NMC Publications.

Pennels C (1999). When is prescribing not prescribing? *NT Nurse Prescribing No 1 09 06 99.* London: Emap Publishing.

Tingle (1998). *Law and Nursing* (with McHale J, Peysner J). Oxford: Butterworth-Heinemann.

Tingle (2002). *Nurses and the Law (Seminar Presentation).* London: Gate House.

Chapter 5

Ethical issues in independent and supplementary prescribing

John Adams

INTRODUCTION

Ethics is concerned with the promotion of the high standards of conduct by which the public rightly expects healthcare practitioners to abide. The relationship between law and ethics in a democratic society should always be a close one. Legislators and judges create laws and legal decisions that can be enforced through the courts. Ethicists, on the other hand, spend their time reflecting on the implications of legal decisions and exploring the ways in which conduct can be guided by rational and coherent principles. There is a constant dialogue between legal scholars and ethicists as each seek to use the other's discipline to shed light on their own concerns, so it is not surprising that most textbooks for the healthcare professions, like this one, combine discussion of both law and ethics.

At the heart of ethics lies the process of reflecting on the dilemmas raised by professional practice. The contribution that ethics makes is to provide a range of possible theoretical tools or frameworks which may help to elucidate the issues that are at stake, and which may provide consistent guidance on which principles should be given the most weight. Ethics does not, therefore, provide a simple system that will provide the 'right' answer when faced with any dilemma in prescribing practice. It is the starting point for the debate rather than its neat and tidy conclusion. Professional practice in healthcare in the modern world requires the balancing of complex competing needs and interests. Practitioners' responses to this kind of ethical exploration and debate depend to a large extent on how useful they feel this process of reflection to be.

The authority to prescribe raises a range of important ethical concerns such as the need to obtain informed consent, the requirement to respect confidentiality, and decisions over the allocation of scarce resources. At the heart of ethical considerations of prescribing is the imbalance of power between the prescriber and the patient. Where one person has power over another, the potential for abuse of that situation always exists, and the power to control access to potentially important medication requires frequent review and reflection.

ETHICAL FRAMEWORKS

Subjective ethics

Many people would argue that ethical decision-making is essentially a simple matter of listening to our conscience. They believe that when confronted with an ethical

47

dilemma, we all know instinctively what the 'right' course of action is. No-one would want to deny the power of conscience. Over the course of many centuries, brave individuals have felt compelled to follow the dictates of their conscience, even at great cost to themselves. Even today, much 'whistle-blowing' activity in the health service is motivated by the subjective guidance of an individual conscience. So while not wishing to diminish the undoubted power of individual subjective approaches to decision-making in ethics, it must also be recognised that it has some serious shortcomings. The fundamental problem posed by subjective approaches to ethics is the potential for lack of consistency, with an absence of agreed principles on which to rely for guidance. If a prescriber announces that they feel free to ignore the requirement for patient confidentiality, or that their conscience tells them to dispense with informed consent, discussion generally proves fruitless. As the saying goes, 'there is no reasoning with conscience'. So while the ability to follow the guidance of conscience is a highly desirable characteristic in any healthcare professional, it is not sufficient on its own. Objective external standards are necessary in order to ensure that practitioners have an outside frame of reference against which to judge their actions.

Paternalism

Paternalism (literally 'acting like a father', by implementing decisions which are felt to be in the patient's best interest, but without obtaining prior informed consent) has been the dominant tradition in Western medicine. Until comparatively recently, healthcare professionals believed that it was their role to decide on courses of treatment without necessarily gaining the consent of the patient. While it is easy to blame the various professions concerned, and to regard paternalism as evidence of an oppressive medical conspiracy, it is probably more correct to see it as expressing the preference of most patients at that time to be told, rather than to be asked. The last 50 years, however, have seen a decisive shift in public opinion against medical paternalism and in favour of informed consent. This fundamental shift in our culture has several roots. Most people now regard decisions about what happens to their own body as among the most important they are ever called upon to take, so they are naturally unwilling to delegate them to health service professionals. Secondly, the dominance of consumerism in all other walks of life has an inevitable impact upon healthcare. As we expect to select from the supermarket precisely what we want, when we want it, it is not surprising that increasingly 'consumerist' attitudes are permeating the health service. Recent scandals involving poor standards of performance by healthcare professionals are only likely to accelerate this trend. Finally, as prescribers are concerned about compliance or concordance with medication regimes, accurate adherence to them is presumably more likely to be achieved if the patient has been fully involved in the decision-making process.

Having outlined some of the shortcomings of traditional medical paternalism, it is important to stress that the opposite extreme, laissez-faire practice, is equally inappropriate. The prescriber who said to all their patients, 'Just tell me what you want and I will prescribe it for you', would not be acting ethically. The prescriber has a responsibility to assess each patient's needs and to recommend a course of treatment, if that is felt to be appropriate. This recommendation will include a willingness to discuss possible side-effects, and the pros and cons of other potential treatment options. In situations where the patient is unable to take part in the decision-making process, because of reduced conscious level or a confused state for example, society would expect a prescriber to make decisions in what are genuinely felt to be the patient's best interest.

Deontological ethics

There is a long tradition of adopting concepts from philosophy in order to illuminate ethical discussion. Deontology (from the Greek word for duty or obligation) is the name given to a school of thought in philosophy which emphasises that there are certain fixed duties which everyone ought to undertake. Most of the great religions of the world promote a deontological approach to ethics. One example, shared by Judaism and Christianity, is the Ten Commandments. The statement 'thou shalt not kill' lays down an ethical standard that does not grant exceptions, or suggest that the consequences of an action in any particular situation should be taken into account. The strength of this kind of approach to ethics is that it encourages all practitioners to aspire to an equally high standard of conduct. Patients can feel confidence that ethical principles will be adhered to whatever the circumstances in which they find themselves. The main weakness, on the other hand, of the deontological approach to ethics is that it is inflexible and may not take particular circumstances into account. To give an extreme example, if a gunman takes a ward full of patients and staff hostage and threatens to kill them all, police marksmen may feel justified in breaking the prohibition against murder in order to save the maximum number of lives. As no healthcare system in the world provides all the resources that every patient may require, healthcare professionals are always faced with the necessity of deciding priorities rather than following unchanging duties. Cash-limited drug budgets present a good example of the kind of prioritisation decisions that have to take place. The prescriber is simply unable to meet every need that could be met.

Immanuel Kant (1724–1804), a professor of philosophy at Königsberg University in Prussia, developed an influential approach to deontological ethics based upon human reason and on religious belief. The central tenet in his approach to ethics is that human beings should always be regarded as ends in themselves, rather than as means to an end. One could imagine a situation in which a pharmaceutical researcher is so convinced that a new drug will benefit humanity that he becomes careless about the sufferings of the people taking part in the drug trials of early versions of the medication. Kant's ethical principle reminds us that all human beings have equal value.

> Immanuel Kant also emphasised that to be ethical, principles should be applicable in all similar situations: he wrote that we should, 'act upon a maxim that can also hold as a universal law'
>
> (Wood, 1999, p. xxi).

When resources are limited, there is always the temptation to make exceptions for special cases: for colleagues, for patients who seem particularly needy or who tug at the heart strings – the list could go on and on. Kant reminds us that fairness and equal rights should lie at the heart of ethically defensible decision-making.

A practitioner with the power to prescribe needs to reflect long and hard about providing something for one person or group that would not normally be available for all.

Utilitarian ethics

In the nineteenth century, leading thinkers turned away from deontological ethics on the grounds that its inflexible rules did not provide guidance for the dilemmas which people face in everyday life. In the place of duty-based ethics, two British philosophers, Jeremy Bentham (1748–1832) and John Stuart Mill (1806–1873) developed a highly influential approach to practical ethics that was based upon the idea of evaluating the consequences of an ethical decision. In their view, the decision that maximised happiness was the ethically correct one to take. The everyday usefulness of this approach was emphasised by their calling it 'utilitarian ethics'. In place of happiness, modern utilitarians tend to advocate decisions that result in 'the greatest good for the greatest number'.

Utilitarian ethics can be found being used to justify actions in all areas of the modern health service. Triage procedures in the accident and emergency department are designed to ensure that patients in most need are treated first. Hospital wards are also generally run on utilitarian principles. Patients deemed to have the greatest clinical need are generally nursed in beds nearest the nurses' station, and receive the most attention. Most countries in the developed world use waiting lists for treatments that give priority to those whose clinical need is judged to be greatest.

In situations where there is agreement about where the 'greatest good' lies, utilitarian ethics command wide acceptance. So most people would agree that the saving of life in the emergency situation takes precedence over other issues. Most people stop their car to allow the ambulance with the blue flashing light to overtake. Similarly, there is a general acceptance that patients with severe trauma should receive priority treatment in the accident and emergency department.

> Utilitarianism provides the classic justification for developing scarce resources to where they will do the greatest good. Drug budgets are finite, while demand is increasing all the time. Yet the word 'rationing' remains firmly off the political agenda. Influential voices the world of pharmaceutical policy have recently called for an open debate on the issue
>
> (Hargreaves, 2003).

The fact that utilitarian justifications are given for decisions taken throughout the health service means that this approach to ethics can soon come to be regarded as 'the obvious way of doing things', and so beyond debate. This makes it particularly important that utilitarianism is not adopted uncritically, and that due weight is given to its potential weaknesses as an ethical philosophy. The main criticism concerns those who lose out when utilitarian criteria are applied. There are losers as well as winners when such judgements are made. Historically, some groups always had a low priority in the competition for scarce National Health Services (NHS) resources – for example, older people, people with a learning disability, and those who were mentally ill. So the question must be posed: what about the needs of the low priority, low status patient? The recent development of an NHS culture of inspections, targets, audit and National Service Frameworks (NSF) can be seen as an attempt to ensure that utilitarian excesses are moderated, and that resources are devoted to all. A second weakness of utilitarian ethics is that it depends upon an ability to predict the future. Indeed, utilitarianism is sometimes referred to as a 'consequentialist' approach to ethics, as the utilitarian must weigh up the likely consequences of possible actions, and choose the option that maximises the happiness or the good. Yet predicting the outcome of a particular clinical decision can be difficult. The continuing development of evidence-based practice should enable practitioners to make more informed judgements about likely outcomes.

Summary

From the perspective of philosophical ethics, the prescriber can be portrayed as trapped between two opposing forces: deontological and utilitarian ethics.

On the one hand, the healthcare professional feels duty bound to meet all the needs that patients present. On the other hand are the pressures exerted by budgetary limits and a health service that often demands that needs are prioritised.

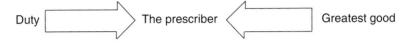

Duty   ⟹   The prescriber   ⟸   Greatest good

A principles-based approach

While deontological and utilitarian approaches to ethics may provide the context in which decisions are taken, practitioners generally feel the need for ethical guidance that is more specifically related to the clinical dilemmas that they face in everyday practice. The most influential figures in the biomedical field are the two American ethicists, Tom L. Beauchamp and James F. Childress. They argue that it is possible to identify four key ethical principles in the medical tradition (respect for autonomy, non-maleficence (that is, avoiding causing harm), beneficence (seeking to do good to patients), and justice), which they supplement with four 'rules', veracity, privacy, confidentiality and fidelity (Beauchamp and Childress, 2001).

Respect for autonomy

It is no co-incidence that Beauchamp and Childress place 'respect for autonomy' first in their consideration of the principles that should guide ethical decision-making. As we have seen, most patients today reject paternalistic attitudes on the part of healthcare professionals. Both the legal and ethical dimensions of informed consent rest on a similar set of procedures. There is an underlying assumption that the patient will have the intellectual capacity to understand the issues that are to be decided, the ability to decide between the various options presented, and a memory of what was decided. The role of the prescriber is to outline the choices to be made, provide sufficient background information including that on any side-effects of the proposed treatment and likely effects of non-treatment, and to recommend a course of action. Even though this approach has become the expected norm, it is easy to find patients who can describe prescribing encounters that have fallen a long way short of this standard.

Recent emphasis on the central importance of obtaining informed consent can sometimes lead practitioners to assume that patients must take part in the decisions concerning their treatment. But if we are serious about respecting autonomy, then presumably we must respect a patient's right not to choose that course of treatment. It is clear that there are some patients who genuinely do not want to take part in such decision-making, and would rather the prescriber acted in their best interest but without their involvement. This is sometimes felt to be a characteristic of some older patients who are believed to be more comfortable with a situation in which 'the prescriber knows best'. However, it is apparent that there are patients of all ages who take such a stance, and respect for their autonomy means that the prescriber should support their choice.

> Consider a scenario in which a patient presents at the clinic with a sore throat and requests a course of antibiotic treatment in order to cure it. After a careful history has been taken, and an examination carried out, the prescriber concludes that a prescription for a course of antibiotic therapy would be inappropriate. The patient says, 'You are just trying to save money from the drug budget'. The prescriber calmly explains the evidence base for the decision. The patient continues to demand a prescription for an antibiotic.

Such is the power of consumerism in our society, with its slogan 'the customer is always right', that some patients have problems in modifying this approach when faced with healthcare settings. Important as 'respect for autonomy' is in current ethical thought, few ethicists would argue that patient choice should override all other considerations. However, while such situations may prove difficult for the current prescriber, the development of information technology looks set to pose even greater challenges in the future. The increasing availability of medical information on the Internet, and the web-based international trade in pharmaceutical products are likely to create major issues for both the individual prescriber and the national regulatory authorities in the not-too-distant future.

In most healthcare settings, and on most occasions, patients follow the advice given to them by the staff. This can soon lead to the complacent belief that 'respect for autonomy' raises few issues. Yet it may only be when a patient makes what the staff consider to be a 'foolish' decision that the concept of autonomy and its limits is fully explored. Our society is gradually becoming more accepting of such patient decisions. Refusing to accept medication may shorten life, but society now generally accepts such a decision in a competent adult.

Non-maleficence
The principle of non-maleficence means that the prescriber has an active duty to avoid causing harm to patients. This concept is sometimes encountered in the form of the Latin phrase, 'primum non nocere' – above all, do no harm – and some clinicians regard it as the central concept in medical ethics. Medication can have seriously harmful consequences, and for some patients may even prove to be fatal. So the prescriber clearly has an ethical duty to consider carefully any harmful effects that the prescribed medication may have. It could therefore be argued that maintaining professional competence through evidence-based practice is an ethical imperative as well as a professional one. However, non-maleficence can never be an absolute requirement as all drugs have potentially harmful side-effects, and a

desire to avoid all harm would inevitably mean that no prescriptions were ever written. So the challenge for the prescriber seeking to prescribe ethically is to judge which risks, and which levels of risk, are appropriate in any given clinical situation.

> The current emphasis on the unwanted side-effects of medication can some-times have an unfortunate influence upon decision-making by patients. I used to visit a sprightly woman of 90, who had a store of vivid memories about the history of local towns and villages. As she had severe hypertension, her general practitioner (GP) had prescribed antihypertensive medication for her. Whenever I visited, she used to show me the leaflet enclosed in the box. She would unroll it like an ancient scroll, and solemnly intone the list of frightening conditions of which she was warned. It did indeed appear that these innocuous-looking tablets threatened just about every ill known to humankind. Being struck by lightening seemed to be just about the only risk not to be increased. So my advice to her to follow the prescriber's instructions fell on deaf ears. When feeling particularly unwell, she took a few of the tablets, but as soon as she started to feel better they were discontinued – 'because they can harm you, dear – just look at what it says in this leaflet!'

Beneficence

Beneficence – the duty to do good – has always been central to the role of the healthcare professional. It is an dynamic process which actively seeks out the most appropriate treatment for the patient. Therefore beneficence is underpinned by regular professional updating so that the most effective therapies can be prescribed. While few would argue with the importance of beneficence when expressed in this way, the risk is that it shades over into paternalism: 'I know what is good for you: trust me, I'm a prescriber'.

Justice

Philosophers since at least the time of Aristotle have argued that human beings have an innate regard for justice. Fairness, however, requires restraint on the part of some who could grab more than their fair share. When drug budgets are limited, the issue of justice towards patients is an important and controversial one. As priorities have to be set, one approach is that local trusts are best placed to distribute their resources in an equitable manner. As this will inevitably mean that a drug or treatment will be available in one area but not another, the campaigning cry immediately goes up that this is 'post-code prescribing'. Both NSF and the National Institute for Clinical Excellence (NICE) have been specifically charged with the task of ensuring uniformity across the NHS. How local priorities and national requirements can be reconciled has yet to be elucidated.

Veracity   Veracity, or truthfulness, is an essential component of informed consent and hence of respect for autonomy. Asking a patient whether they would choose the red tablets or the purple ones, without further information, does not show respect for autonomy. While everyone supports the principle of veracity, putting it into practice provides major scope for ethical dilemmas. Issues around how much should be told, to whom, and in what circumstances, creates continuing difficulty for healthcare professionals. As we saw earlier, complete information on side-effects may cause the patient to stop taking the medication. But who is to say what is 'enough'? Even starker dilemmas are raised if bad news is to be conveyed.

Privacy   Elevating the concept of privacy to a key role in ethical debate represents a new and challenging departure from the traditions of medical ethics. The key issue here is what information should a patient share with a healthcare professional, and what can be kept secret. The concept of patient privacy forms a thought-provoking challenge to some current concepts of 'holistic assessment and care planning'. Ranging across the 'twelve activities of living' (Roper *et al.*, 2000) to collect information about a patient's lifestyle far removed from the presenting problem, may have major implications for the desire for privacy. Even though the NHS has in the past set little store by patient privacy in its communal wards and clinics, some areas of privacy have existed for many years. One example is treatment in a clinic for sexually transmitted diseases. The records of such treatment episodes are kept separate from general hospital records, and so patients' privacy is maintained if treatment is sought for other types of condition. Such a system operates effectively when paper records are involved, but increasing automation poses real threats to privacy. The development of an electronic patient record needs to take such concerns into account if it is to command public trust (Mandl *et al.*, 2001).

Confidentiality   Modern medical treatment almost always requires communication of patient details between departments, teams and individuals, if the optimum level of care is to be provided. This immediately undermines the old ideal of patient secrets being retained by one doctor. So health service organisations must continually review their measures in place to protect patient confidentiality.

Fidelity   Fidelity is concerned with faithfully maintaining the duty to care, even in difficult circumstances. The NHS and its staff has a generally laudable tradition of maintaining treatment for patients or clients who have been stigmatised or even rejected by the rest of society. A local television news programme recently reported on the plight of a group of traveller families in great need, from whom all contacts with official bodies had been withdrawn. The only 'professional' who continued to offer support was a health visitor. Her on-going care for the children and their parents demonstrated fidelity in action. Prescribers are likely to have frequent contact with patients who exhibit challenging behaviour, or who are stigmatised for some reason. Possession of the power of control over medication inevitably places the prescriber on society's 'front line'. The concept of fidelity provides a reminder of society's expectation of the manner in which the power is to be exercised.

Codes of Conduct

One of the earliest statements of ethical principles in medicine was the Hippocratic oath. Like all ethical codes, it combines timeless precepts with ideas relevant only to the time and society that created it. It advocates doing good and avoiding harm, and not taking advantage of the vulnerable, but it also forbids doctors from undertaking surgical procedures. This reflects a historical context in which educated physicians looked down upon the artisans who combined the practice of surgery with blood-letting and maintaining a barber's shop. Many of the Hippocratic precepts, such as 'doing good' and 'avoiding harm', can still be found in modern

Codes of Conduct for healthcare professionals. The principles-based approach of Beauchamp and Childress (2001) has also been highly influential in the development of such codes. One example is the Code of Professional Conduct of the Nursing and Midwifery Council (2002). Many of its clauses can be mapped against their principles and rules. For example:

- Respect for autonomy:
  - Section 2: As a registered nurse or midwife, you must respect the patient or client as an individual.
  - Section 3: As a registered nurse or midwife, you must obtain consent before you give any treatment or care.

- Non-maleficence:
  - Section 8: As a registered nurse or midwife, you must act to identify and minimise the risk to patients and clients.

- Beneficence:
  - Section 1.4: You have a duty of care to your patients and clients, who are entitled to receive safe and competent care.

- Justice:
  - Section 2.2: You are personally accountable for ensuring that you promote and protect the interests and dignity of patients and clients, irrespective of gender, age, race, ability, sexuality, economic status, lifestyle, culture and religious or political beliefs.

- Veracity:
  - Section 3.1: Information should be accurate, truthful and presented in such a way as to make it easily understood.

- Confidentiality:
  - Section 5: As a registered nurse or midwife, you must protect confidential information.

- Fidelity:
  - Section 7: As a registered nurse or midwife, you must be trustworthy.

A similar exercise can be carried out with the Code of Ethics and Standards published by the Royal Pharmaceutical Society of Great Britain (2003), which can be downloaded from their website (http://www.rpsgb.org.uk).

The prescriber and the pharmaceutical companies

The attainment of prescribing rights will inevitably bring the individual prescriber into close contact with the pharmaceutical companies and their representatives. The ethical aspects of existing links between the industry and medical practitioners are widely debated. Some argue that doctors need to 'disentangle' themselves from this relationship, while others advocate a continuing dialogue between the two parties (Moynihan, 2003a, b; Wager, 2003). In the UK, the activities of pharmaceutical companies are subject to the Association of the British Pharmaceutical Industry (ABPI) Code of Practice for the Pharmaceutical Industry (2003), and all prescribers need to familiarise themselves with its provisions.

What is your opinion of this advertisement?

> **Are you a prescriber?**
> **In need of some winter sunshine?**
>
> If you can answer 'YES' to these two questions,
> let Whamo Pharmaceuticals whisk you
> and your partner to a 5-star hotel in
> Monaco
> for a short product briefing
> (… then shop 'til you drop!)

Clause 19.1 of the ABPI Code of Practice for the Pharmaceutical Industry, governing meetings and hospitality, is relevant here. It states that:

- 'hospitality must be secondary to the purpose of the meeting';
- 'the level of hospitality must be appropriate and not out of proportion to the occasion';
- 'the costs involved must not exceed that level which the recipients would normally adopt when paying for themselves';
- '(hospitality) must not extend beyond members of the health professions or appropriate staff'.

As, on the face of it, this advertisement appears to offer hospitality that contravenes all four elements of the clause, referral to the Prescription Medicines Code of Practice Authority would seem to be appropriate.

While attention inevitably tends to focus on those isolated instances when the Code is disregarded, the reality is that pharmaceutical companies make a major contribution to educational activities of all kinds. Attendance at local educational meetings, which may receive sponsorship from pharmaceutical companies, can provide an important source of information about developments in prescribing. The following advertisement appears to indicate a worthwhile meeting with an appropriate level of hospitality.

> **'Current trends in asthma care'**
>
> **Lunchtime lecture**
> **by**
> **Professor M. Fulbourn FRCP**
>
> Location: The Interchange Motel, Loamstone
>
> *Sandwich lunch provided*
> *Sponsors: Whamo Pharmaceuticals*

When the ethics of a prescriber receiving gifts or hospitality from a pharmaceutical company are discussed, attention tends to focus upon any potential influence that this may have upon the behaviour and attitudes of the prescriber. Yet surely this is to ignore the most important participant in the encounter: the patient. Little research has been done on the attitudes of patients towards prescribers receiving gifts from the pharmaceutical industry. In one American study, a survey was conducted to compare the attitudes of prescribing physicians with those of patients attending their hospitals, on whether it was appropriate to accept gifts and whether this would be likely to influence prescribing behaviour (Gibbons *et al.*, 1998). The results indicated that patients found gifts less appropriate and more influential than did their physicians. As the legal profession discovered many years ago: 'justice must not only be done, it must be seen to be done'. Transparency is a key requirement in decision-making processes if the public is to retain confidence in those decisions. In exactly the same way, a prescriber needs to be constantly reviewing how patients may perceive his or her acceptance of gifts.

Picture the scene. You are a patient arriving at a clinic for a consultation. Once inside the consulting room, the first thing you notice is that the handsome desk set and blotter carry a slogan from Whamo Pharmaceuticals. As your eyes rove around the room, you cannot help noticing that the same logo is also displayed on the year planner on the wall, and on the prescriber's smart document case lying on the floor. Having assessed your condition thoroughly, the healthcare professional explains that you need a prescription for the new drug, Whamo-lite. As the pen (guess who provided it!) moves effortlessly across the prescription pad, how much confidence do you feel in the independence of the prescriber's judgement?

Research ethics and the prescriber

Pharmaceutical research is a major generator of the research activity in the NHS, and much of it involves the crucial participation of prescribers, so prescribers need to be aware of the main features of the NHS system in place to review research protocols in order to provide ethical safeguards for patients and staff. The cornerstone of the system is the Local Research Ethics Committee (LREC), which regulates research within a defined geographical area. LRECs were first established in the 1960s, and their procedures were set out in health service guidance published in 1991 (HSG (91) 5). Originally, the area covered by a LREC was relatively small, and so major studies conducted by pharmaceutical companies required detailed negotiations with numerous LRECs. In 1997, a new tier of regulation for large studies, the Multi-Centre REC (MREC) was set up (HSG (97) 23). Policy in the area of research ethics is currently guided by the document Governance Arrangements for NHS RECs (2001), but the implementation of its requirements has been a gradual process, and at the time of writing this chapter (September 2003) the process of transition is still on-going. The co-ordination of this process in England is being undertaken by a new organisation, the Central Office for RECs (CORECs), which maintains an informative website (http://www.corec.org.uk). Similar initiatives are being undertaken in Wales, Scotland and Northern Ireland.

The COREC working on behalf of the Department of Health (DoH) in England:

- Co-ordinates the development of operational systems for LRECs and MRECs on behalf of the NHS in England.

- Maintains an overview of the operations of the research ethics system in England, and alerts the DoH and other responsible authorities if the need arises for them to review policy and operational guidance relating to RECs.

- Manages the MRECs in England.

- Develops and manages a national training programme for REC members and administrators in England.

- Maintains close contact with officials in the DoH with policy responsibility for wider issues of research ethics and with colleagues from Scotland, Wales and Northern Ireland.

- With appropriate advice, develops, implements and maintains operating procedures and standards for RECs that will be consistent across the UK.

- Establishes and manages regional Offices of RECs (ORECs) to oversee the activity of LRECs.

- Provides advice to the DoH on the implications and practicalities of transposing the EU Directive on Good Clinical Practice in Medicinal Trials in the UK.

From the COREC website

The guiding principle in research ethics is that 'the dignity, rights, safety and well being of participants must be the primary consideration' (DoH, 2001).

Ethical advice from the appropriate NHS REC is required for any research proposal involving:

- Patients and users of the NHS. This includes all potential research participants recruited by virtue of the patient or user's past or present treatment by, or use of, the NHS. It includes NHS patients treated under contracts with private sector institutions.

- Individuals identified as potential research participants because of their status as relatives or carers of patients and users of the NHS, as defined above.

- Access to data, organs or other bodily material of past and present NHS patients.

- Fetal material and in vitro fertilisation (IVF) involving NHS patients.

- The recently dead in NHS premises.

- The use of, or potential access to, NHS premises or facilities.

- NHS staff – recruited as research participants by virtue of their professional role.

DoH (2001)

CONCLUSION

All medical scandals tend to result in calls for ever-tighter regulation of healthcare professionals, and for more emphasis to be placed on the teaching of ethics. Then when there is a great national outcry over the misuse of medication for criminal purposes – the cases of nurse Beverley Allitt and Dr Harold Shipman are examples – the cry inevitably goes up from the mass media: 'healthcare professionals must have more teaching on ethics'. No amount of reflection on ethics, however, is likely to have stopped those who have such murderous inclinations. In addition, when such stories break, calls are inevitably made for the closer supervision of prescribers. While there is no doubt some merit in reviewing the regulations, there are finite limits to what such supervision can achieve. In the final analysis, society has no alternative but to trust prescribers (O'Neill, 2002). So the responsibility for fostering that trust lies with all who have the authority to prescribe.

References

Association of British Pharmaceutical Industries (2003). ABPI Code of Practice for the Pharmaceutical Industry. (http://www.abpi.org.uk/publications/pdfs/codeofpractise03.pdf)

Beauchamp TL, Childress JF (2001). *Principles of Biomedical Ethics* 5th edn. New York: Oxford University Press.

Department of Health (2001). *Governance Arrangements for NHS Research Ethics Committees.* London: DoH.

Gibbons RV, Landry FJ, Blouch DL, Jones DL, Williams FK, Lucey CR, Kroenke K (1998). A comparison of physicians' and patients' attitudes toward pharmaceutical industry gifts. *Journal of General Internal Medicine* **13**: 151–154.

Hargreaves S (2003). News: transparency is key to rationing, delegates told. *British Medical Journal* **326**: 619.

Mandl KD, Szolovits P, Kohane IS (2001). Public standards and patients' control: how to keep electronic medical records accessible but private. *British Medical Journal* **322**: 283–286.

Moynihan R (2003a). Who pays for the pizza? Redefining the relationships between doctors and drug companies. 1: Entanglement. *British Medical Journal* **326**: 1189–1192.

Moynihan R (2003b). Who pays for the pizza? Redefining the relationships between doctors and drug companies. 2: Disentanglement. *British Medical Journal* **326**: 1193–1196.

Nursing and Midwifery Council (2002). *Code of Professional Conduct.* London: Nursing and Midwifery Council.

O'Neill O (2002). *Autonomy and Trust in Bioethics.* Cambridge: Cambridge University Press.

Roper N, Logan WW, Tierney AJ (2000). *The Roper–Logan–Tierney Model of Nursing: Based on Activities of Living.* Edinburgh: Churchill Livingstone.

Royal Pharmaceutical Society (2003). Code of Ethics and Standards. (http://www.rpsgb.org.uk/pdfs/MEP27s2.pdf).

Wager E (2003). How to dance with porcupines: rules and guidelines on doctors' relations with drug companies. *British Medical Journal* **326**: 1196–1198.

Wood AW (1999). *Kant's Ethical Thought.* Cambridge: Cambridge University Press.

Chapter 6

Psychology and sociology of prescribing

Tom Walley and Robin Williams

INTRODUCTION

Why do doctors and other health professionals prescribe medicines? Why do patients want to take medicines? The simple answers to these questions can all be framed in terms of a biomedical model of the patient presenting with an illness and the prescriber trying to provide the means to help the patient get better. But this is only a partial truth, and in reality, prescribing is a more complex social interaction. Prescribing can be a means to a variety of ends. Unless we understand this, and understand why prescribers and patients behave as they do, we cannot understand prescribing. What is termed 'irrational prescribing' can often be explained, and by this understanding, we can work towards helping both prescribers and patients make the best use of medicines.

This chapter concerns itself with the multiplicity of non-biomedical reasons why patients may or may not receive a prescription. These lie partly in the psychology of the interaction between the individual prescriber and patient, but partly in the societies or cultures (professional, ethnic, local or even national) within which each operates; these two are so interwoven that they are best considered side-by-side.

In this chapter, we will talk a lot about doctor behaviour. This is because almost all of the research so far is about how doctors, rather than other professionals, behave in relation to prescribing. But the reasons why doctors prescribe are the same as those which will drive the prescribing of other professions, and to assume that nurses or pharmacists will prescribe better, or be less influenced by these pressures because they spend longer with the patient and so won't fall into all of the problems discussed here, is simply false.

SOCIOLOGICAL MODELS

It might help to give a description of various medical sociological theories or models that have been developed to explain prescribing behaviour.

Lay belief system

Nurses, doctors, pharmacists and many healthcare professionals have beliefs firmly lodged in what can be termed 'Western modern medicine' – a belief in medicine as a science rather than a superstition, in the principles of evidence-based medicine, in physical rather than magical causes for illness, and conversely in pharmacological cures rather than placebo. But people, namely most patients, work outside this close-knit professional group and have widely differing ideas. These ideas do not fit neatly into the scientific belief system. The range of these ideas is quite staggering and varies significantly among social groups within different cultures. These beliefs strongly determine when patients seek medical care, their expectations about receiving medicines and the type of treatments that they seek.

The sick role

This was first described by Talcott Parsons back in 1951. The sick role is deemed a temporary state wherein the patient cedes control of his life to others, usually to medics and nurses, on the grounds of ill health. This may be some form of global ill health requiring, for instance, hospital admission, or a much narrower role, such as high blood pressure. The person then becomes a patient, who is expected to accept and follow the advice of these professionals. At the same time, an individual who enters the sick role then becomes privileged and protected, and is then able to shed some of their responsibilities such as the need to go to work or turn up for school.

Sanctioning and legitimising

Doctors have traditionally acted as gatekeepers into this sick role, but increasingly professionals other than doctors are also involved. For many patients, a prescription is the ticket for entry into or to confirm this role. It is the external legitimisation of some illnesses, and conversely if a doctor refuses a prescription, friends or relatives may assume 'there's nothing much wrong with him' i.e. the legitimisation has been denied. For many patients, it is as if the doctor has refused to acknowledge their illness. The patient may therefore be very resentful of such a refusal, and the prescriber may not be well accepted by the patient when trying to explain for instance that antibiotics do not work for viral illnesses.

Doctors act as gatekeepers not only to medical care, but also to many aspects of social care. Doctors enable people to take time off work or not go to school. They may enable access to sick pay or other benefits. Society tends to define the boundaries, and a patient whom the doctor deems unfit for these privileges might be considered a malingerer. This is a very powerful position for the professions. Prescribing might be one expression of sanctioning this process.

Medicalisation

More and more areas seem to become subject to the control and the jurisdiction of medicine. Doctors and other may encourage this to extend their professional power. The medical supervision of the natural act of childbirth or the menopause might be seen as examples of this. People such as Illich (1981) (author of the famous book, *Medical Nemesis*) believe this whole process has gone too far.

Prescribing responsibility is an expression of this power. Drugs may become part of this medicalisation, as the pharmaceutical industry seeks new markets to extend its profits. For instance is a disease increasingly defined by the fact that there is a drug available to treat the problem? This is perhaps most apparent when we think about so called 'lifestyle drugs' such as sildenafil (Viagra) or orlistat (Xenical) (Gilbert *et al.*, 2000). While recognising that obesity is a serious problem that causes a lot of morbidity, when does it move from a matter of personal choice (to eat too much; to exercise too little) to a medical matter in which the patient cedes control to the professionals? To what extent did this develop when there were drugs available to treat the condition? There is no easy answer to this question, which is often rooted in cultural perceptions of what is illness. For instance, the French consume vast amounts of medication (about 55 prescriptions per head per year), while the Dutch take very little by comparison (around five to six prescriptions per year). In the UK, the average is 11–12 per year. This is not explained by the French being vastly more unhealthy than the Dutch, and clearly the French have a different idea about what is appropriate medical care.

Opposing this growing medicalisation is a counterculture of patients becoming more assertive in taking more control of their own health and being involved in their own treatments. The chapter on concordance will say much more about this. There is clearly a balance to be struck here between self care and care from health professionals, and the balance varies from culture to culture, and from patient to patient.

WHY DO DOCTORS (AND OTHERS) PRESCRIBE?

As we said in the introduction, this question could be answered simply in a biomedical way about illness, the pathophysiology of the illness and a desire to use the pharmacological effect of a drug to improve the patient's condition. Harris and co-workers (1990) describe this as the 'respectable' answer, but found a lot of evidence that doctors often prescribe even when they anticipate no real medical benefit from the drug. They identify a range of non-biomedical reasons why doctors prescribe:

- *To avoid doing something else*: for example, like referring a patient to hospital or another service.

- *To maintain contact*: This may seem to be an odd point but remember that a general practitioner (GP) has to work with a patient to improve the patient's health over many years. If he antagonises a patient over a refused prescription for an antibiotic, the relationship may fail and undermine what the doctor might want to do about long-term management of the patient's diabetes or ischaemic heart disease. In this situation, many doctors would let the occasional (biomedically 'inappropriate') prescription pass. This is not an excuse for prescribing anything to everyone, as again there has to be a balance. The occasional prescription in this way may leave the door open for the patient to return with the same or other problems, while a cold refusal of a prescription may seem to slam the door in the patient's face.

- *To temporise and gain time*: Often the diagnosis is not clear in early disease. So prescribing may allow time for the disease process to become clear or if it is a self-limiting illness, to go away. This temporising is part of the first two points – to avoid referring the patient perhaps needlessly, while keeping the process under observation. It may also be important to allow patients time to understand their own diseases or conditions.

For some doctors, this is a way of dealing with uncertainty: in general practice in particular, the diagnosis is often unclear and the doctor responds to her 'best formulation' of what is wrong with the patient and acts accordingly. Some doctors find such uncertainty very difficult, and handle it by making firm (but sometimes unwarranted) diagnoses, and then prescribing.

- *To satisfy an urge to give*: The patient has come to the doctor with some distress. There may be a very human feeling that the doctor has to give something to the patient out of compassion, even if what is given is inappropriate. A doctor may see a single mother with two children living on the twelfth floor of a high-rise tower block where vandalism means the lifts are often out of action. The patient might complain of anxiety and depression, and who might not be anxious or depressed in such circumstances? Prescribing anything may be considered inappropriate – this is after all not a medical, but a social problem. Nevertheless, the human urge to support the patient in some way and not reject the patient's distress may lead to a prescription for an anxiolytic or an antidepressant. There may even be some rationalising as to the reasons why the prescription was written, so that it apparently fits into the respectable biomedical model.

The ability to empathise with the patient may be a key factor here. In one study, Howie (1976) showed doctors pictures of a sore throat with a brief vignette of the patient and clinical circumstances, and asked the doctors whether they would prescribe antibiotics or not. In fact the pictures and the vignettes were randomly paired and it was not the clinical features which determined the decision to prescribe but factors such as time of day, previous experience with this particular patient, and often the social standing of the patient (more likely to prescribe an antibiotic for the child of a barrister than a labourer). We have conducted informal studies in the same way with nurses and pharmacists: those who were mothers were particularly given to prescribing for children, and the younger subjects were particularly keen to prescribe for a vignette that involved a young student coming up to examinations. So when the potential prescriber empathised with the patient's situation, it elicited a prescription more easily.

Others have expanded this list of reasons for prescribing considerably and some of these suggestions are even further removed from the 'respectable':

- To terminate the consultation (how often do some doctors reach for the prescription pad as soon as the patient walks in the door?).

- To maintain the role of the doctor (is this being undermined by increasing availability of over the counter drugs and nurse or pharmacist prescribing?).

- To use the power of the placebo effect (see below).

- To legitimise the patient's illness, as we have talked about above.

- To earn money in pharmaceutical industry sponsored post-marketing surveillance studies.

- To avoid medicolegal fears, as a feature of defensive medicine ('I might be sued if I don't prescribe an antibiotic here and something terrible, however rare or unlikely, happens').

- To avoid being called out (or paying for the deputising service). This is said to be the reason for a lot of Friday afternoon antibiotic prescriptions when the doctor prescribes because he won't be available to monitor the condition of the patient over the weekend. There is an element of peer pressure here for the doctor – who may fear criticism from colleagues if they get called out to deal with a deteriorating patient over a weekend.

- Habit or previous experience – we are all heavily influenced by what happened the last time we did something or prescribed something. If a patient had a severe adverse effect we are not going to prescribe *that* drug again no matter how rare the adverse reaction is.

- Precedent ('Dr X always prescribes drug Y for me when I have this ...').

And so on ... you could think of lots more reasons from your personal observations or practice.

Is prescribing for these non-medical reasons, or allowing your decision to prescribe be influenced by any of these, rational? From a strict biomedical standpoint perhaps not, but from many other points it might be. Again there is a balance to be struck here. For most of us, the balance we would like to achieve lies heavily but not exclusively on the biomedical side. But we cannot ignore the other reasons for prescribing and should reflect honestly on our own practice to consider where our point of balance is. Perhaps the worst position is to fool ourselves that we are always acting on the biomedical side when in fact we are responding to other pressures.

Sometimes we rationalise these influences and create more legitimate reasons for prescribing, and often it is not black and white, any more than diagnoses are – these influences may play their biggest role when the biomedical decision to prescribe or not prescribe is marginal, rather than when to prescribe at all would be thought inappropriate. But the doctor who tells himself that he is prescribing antibiotics for what he knows are viral infections 'in case of a bacterial superinfection' is deluding himself – in effect prescribing a dual placebo, both for the patient and for himself.

OTHER INFLUENCES ON THE DOCTOR

We will look at the patient's influence on the doctor later but to be complete, we need to consider some other influences directly on the doctor outside the consultation (Bradley, 1990).

- *Colleagues*: Senior colleagues ('opinion leaders') are very influential in encouraging the issuing of a prescription or not in particular circumstances – medical teachers have particular responsibilities here. Peer pressure is a very important factor, as most of us do not like to be too out of line with what everyone else is doing. This factor is often used either by pharmaceutical companies or by health authorities to influence prescribing.

- *Pharmaceutical companies* are very influential, both for good and for bad. They can be a valuable source of education for many doctors but it has to be remembered that their role is to make profits by encouraging more use of their products. For instance there are many non-steroidal anti-inflammatory drugs advertised for osteoarthritis but none of these advertisements ever describe their drug as being best reserved for patients who fail to respond to non-pharmacological treatments or to paracetamol. In preventing stroke, the thiazide diuretics are inexpensive and no drug has ever been shown to be superior, yet this is omitted from advertisements of newer, more costly drugs for blood pressure. Finally, advertisements always portray a good outcome and fail to mention the often not insubstantial risk of serious adverse effects. The content of this advertising is therefore often biased.

The key weapon in selling drugs is however the pharmaceutical representative who is carefully trained in selling techniques. Not the least of these is giving small presents like pens etc. The point of these gifts is several fold – it creates a desire to reciprocate (by prescribing the representative's product), and it puts a reminder of the name of the product in front of the doctor. The representative is the most expensive part of the industry's portfolio of promotion but also the most powerful – in effect engaging in a 'consultation' with the doctor, and having the face-to-face opportunity to negotiate a satisfactory (to the company) endpoint.

The industry invests heavily in promotion – one estimate from several years ago valued this at £10,000 per doctor per year and it is probably substantially more than this now. The industry might argue that the promotion only encourages the choice of product, i.e. the decision what to prescribe rather than whether to prescribe at all, but this is a direct parallel with the tobacco industry which argued that cigarette advertising might only encourage people to change brand but not to smoke where otherwise they would not. This argument in relation to cigarette advertising is now rejected of course, and it seems reasonable to assume that part of the role of promotion of pharmaceuticals is to encourage prescribing where it would not have otherwise happened. Some of this may be appropriate, for example, where patients have been undertreated, but some of it is not and may lead to over use of medicines in places where fewer or even no drugs should be used. A key target for the representatives is the 'innovator', the doctor who wants to try everything new (but who is also fickle and who will drop the drug as soon as something new comes along). This doctor will help the representative get a foot in the door to win over the more conservative local doctors ('Dr X is prescribing our new drug now, don't you think you should try it too?'). From there, the drug spreads into the 'early adoptors' who are slower to take it up but more likely to stick with it, then the 'late adopters' and finally the 'laggards'.

So does promotion lead to less rational prescribing? It is difficult to study this but it is clear that doctors who prescribe less rationally (i.e. more expensively when lower cost alternatives were available, and with higher rates of prescribing) are more likely to be those who meet with a lot of representatives; but it is hard to say which is the chicken and which the egg. Does the doctor prescribe more because he sees more representatives or is it the other way around?

There is an important point here for non-medical prescribers: pharmaceutical companies find it more and more difficult to access doctors, and most doctors, if only by experience, have some degree of cynicism with regard to the biased messages of the industry. Companies now clearly feel that non-medical prescribers – perhaps nurses more than pharmacists – are a good alternative target for their activities, with responsibilities for prescribing, and for influencing colleagues and perhaps a little naïve. Good advice on how to manage the representatives was provided by the Drugs and Therapeutics Bulletin some years ago (Anon, 1983).

- *The National Health Service (NHS)*: Since most of us want to support the broader aims of the NHS, efforts by the NHS to influence our prescribing are particularly powerful psychological and social influences on us to prescribe in certain ways. GPs have prescribing budgets to remind them of the costs of what they prescribe, set by the primary care trusts; and primary care trusts and hospitals are also responsibile for the clinical governance of the care they provide including prescribing. They will therefore try to improve the quality of prescribing while containing costs as much as possible. They will do this in a variety of ways: professionally by education, newsletters, peer support or pressure, and managerially by budget setting, negotiations with hospitals or other providers, and by configuring other services (e.g. how many nurse-independent prescribers (IP) or supplementary prescribers (SP) they need, and where). There is a range of other NHS resources to support prescribing – these are outlined in other chapters. One of the key aims of these services is to help us to translate the research evidence of how best to treat patients into practice – often a tall order, and outside the remit of this chapter.

PLACEBOS

A placebo (Latin: 'I will please') is an inert or inactive substance or a sham procedure knowingly prescribed or undertaken, not for its specific pharmacological or physiological effect, but for its non-specific psychological or psycho-physiological therapeutic effect. The importance of these effects was often underplayed in the past. The development of the randomised controlled trial showed the true power of this effect. For instance, in mild depression, the response to a supposedly therapeutic drug might be 70% (a doctor who prescribed such a drug might feel very satisfied that he can take credit for such a satisfactory outcome) – but the response to a placebo in the same trial can be as high as 60%. This reflects in part the natural history of the condition (most patients get better whatever you do) but also the ability of the placebo to bring about a physical improvement by influencing the patient's expectations and hopes. Some feel that the use of a placebo is unethical, as it is basically lying to a patient (albeit, in a stark example of medical paternalism, for the patient's own good). Nevertheless all doctors recognise the effects of reassurance to a patient, and acknowledging the patient's distress in some way, and all use this placebo effect to some degree. In Britain, there are no legally prescribable placebos, and sometimes patients are prescribed what might be harmless drugs such as water-soluble vitamins. However, we also use more powerful drugs like antibiotics in this way, and then claim the credit. This has disadvantages: it puts the patient at the risk of potentially serious adverse effects, it is fundamentally dishonest and may undermine the prescriber patient relationship, and may even lead to us deluding ourselves.

There is also a *nocebo* ('I will harm') effect when an innocuous substance apparently produces adverse effects – this is seen in most clinical trials to some degree where a 'placebo' is used. So these psychological influences can work either way depending on how they are communicated to a patient.

The placebo effect is very important and underestimated. We should use it with caution and as rarely as possible, depending instead on honest reassurance and information to the patient. But there are times when we should use this effect knowingly and without deceiving ourselves.

SO WHY DO PATIENTS WANT PRESCRIPTIONS?

This is of course the other side of the coin. Perhaps to start with, the key question is:

- Do patients actually want a prescription?

Research seems to suggest prescribers tend to over-rate the patient's expectation of a prescription (though perhaps not by as much as was previously thought – see below). Indeed the public are often averse to wanting drugs – something that the professionals often overlook. Some patients will refuse prescriptions, either directly or indirectly by simply not getting the prescription filled or not taking the tablets. Concordance addresses many of these issues.

PATIENT PRESSURE

Another factor is what doctors perceive as patient pressure for prescriptions. Some doctors believe that patients are never satisfied without a prescription, and act accordingly. Harris categorised this as 'avoidance' because it is in effect an avoidance of the alternative strategy of spending more time with patients to clarify their views and the nature of their problems.

Is there evidence of a great and unreasonable desire for medication from patients? How reasonable is it for doctors to put the blame for the increased volume of prescribing over the past two decades onto 'patient pressure'? Some reject the concept of patient pressure, and argue that patients' views are more involved, with beliefs about medicines being more complex than 'wants an antibiotic'.

Britten and co-workers (2002) conducted semi-structured interviews with 30 adults and later more extensive questionnaires with several hundred adults to reveal their attitudes to medicines. Patients held a variety of views, some of which might be considered 'orthodox' and others 'unorthodox'. The orthodox views held might be considered medically legitimate, and they relate to a positive view of medicines, taken for a broadly biomedical reason, and with a high expectation for a prescription. Other patients held more unorthodox views, in which there were powerful negative views about medicines and their adverse effects, a feeling that at least some doctors over-prescribed and a low desire and expectation for a prescription. The key point was that many patients held both orthodox and unorthodox views simultaneously, and were very ambivalent about their medicines and medicine taking – on the one hand recognising that the medicines were for their own benefit, on the other hand that medicines can cause adverse effects and wanting to reject perhaps the whole sick role. It is little wonder that compliance with medicines is so poor and concordance so difficult to achieve.

When GPs are surveyed, they often describe high levels of demand for prescriptions, but objective evidence consistently suggests that doctors overestimate patients' expectations. Early studies suggested that many patients interviewed in waiting rooms claimed to want advice or reassurance only, at least as often as a prescription. More recent studies in inner city areas suggest that the figure is as high as 67% wanting a prescription – particularly high in patients who were exempt from prescription charges, and older patients. There is evidence that the doctor responds to what they perceive to be patient expectation (whether this is real or not), even when the doctor thinks that a prescription is not strictly medically necessary.

In one study (McFarlane *et al.*, 1997), 76 GPs recorded clinical data, their certainty about their prescribing decision and any influences on that decision in 1014 consecutively previously well adults suffering with lower respiratory infection. The patients did a similar exercise. Most patients believed that bacterial infection was the problem, antibiotics were the answer, and expected a prescription. The doctors thought that antibiotics were not indicated in many of these patients but were often influenced to prescribe nevertheless by the patients' expectations. Patients who expected an antibiotic but did not receive one were twice as likely to re-consult as those who did not expect an antibiotic, although their clinical outcomes were no worse.

A key issue here is the quality of the doctor's consultation skills, and how well the doctor negotiates a therapeutic contract with the patient. Longer consultations can reduce prescribing rates but if the consultation goes on too long, prescribing rates increase again as all kinds of hidden agendas/diagnoses start to appear.

We should therefore be working to help prescribers and patient talk to one another more clearly and this is a key aim of concordance.

REASONS FOR WANTING A PRESCRIPTION

Many reasons and motives have been described. Some of these include:

1. The patient perceives therapeutic effect for themselves or others. This is almost a biomedical type belief in the power of medicines, which may not be in line with the professionals' more scientific beliefs on this point of course. There are also sometimes elements of superstition around the power of the prescription. This is discussed more under 'health beliefs' below.

2. To avoid expenditure (e.g. a prescription for Calpol for a child rather than buying it from a pharmacy perhaps?)

3. To sanction or make contact with the doctor

4. To achieve recognition of the sick role and to legitimise time off work or school

5. Suggestion by an opinion leader (e.g. mother or friend, etc.)

6. Because it repeats a previous experience (see below about sore throats as an example of this)

7. To receive a 'gift' from the doctor. Many patients end up taking drugs they perhaps did not really want or need because they don't want to reject the doctor's advice or her human response to the patient's distress.

And so on ...

HEALTH BELIEFS

The health beliefs of patients are determined by many factors, many of which are 'cultural'. Attitudes to medicines seem to vary between nations and even among communities within the same nation. The origins of these beliefs are difficult to establish, but it is clear that many are based in myth and legend, and are centuries old. Others develop within a short time, influenced by public opinion, the media, and perhaps by information derived from authoritarian or scientific expert sources. Even the latter beliefs, arising in recent years, are often firmly rooted in myth and image. Is Viagra the answer to unsatisfactory sexual relationships? Is Orlistat a solution to obesity?

These influences are passed on by comment on others' personal experience, in jokes, in learned debates, in the media of all types (often with pharmaceutical industry influence), and by one's own experience of what seems to be important, what seems to work, and what doesn't. The intangible nature of the whole process stems in part from the fact that for most people, the strongest influences on their own beliefs are the images that are passed on by those near to us. Only rarely will those images be based on any controlled or scientifically evaluated experience. Many of the beliefs become self-fulfilling prophecies, or superstitions, which take an increasingly secure hold despite the weakness of their origins.

An important question arises about the power of experience to influence these beliefs. If an average person is offered an antibiotic for a cold or a sore throat by a doctor for whom they have respect, what happens to their readiness to seek antibiotics in the future? Will they dismiss the experience as perhaps not fitting in with what they have learned from other doctors in the rest of their lifetime, or will they change their views because of that act, and because no great adversity has affected them subsequently?

Such an experiment was performed in Southampton (Little *et al.*, 1997). The original idea of the study was to perform a randomised controlled trial to see if the strategy of giving antibiotics for sore throat only when it was essential as defined by very firm medical criteria, or a more liberal attitude to routine use of antibiotics for sore throats regularly, made an important clinical difference to outcomes (it did not). But what was noticed was that the patients who received the antibiotics were, as a group, more likely to return for antibiotics if they suffered a further episode of sore throat, and they were more positively oriented towards antibiotics than those who never received them, even though at the end of the day these patient were no better for having received the antibiotic. These patients had been 'taught' that antibiotics were the appropriate response to a sore throat.

RACE AND CULTURE

Some health beliefs go deeper and seem to be engrained in some specific cultures. In prescribing, it is important to have some understanding of transcultural issues and how these will affect how patient view the prescription and the need for a medicine. Some ethnic minorities tend to have fixed views about this. In some cultures, disease is seen as always something external to the patient and must therefore be fought off with external aid such as a prescription medicine. In some ethnic minorities, a mother who did not bring her child to the doctor at the first sign of an infection would be considered a bad parent. By follow on, a doctor who does not prescribe (and legitimise the whole process) may lose contact with the family who may avoid her in the future. These pressures can be subtle and require an awareness and sensitivity on the part of the prescriber. Sometimes they are less subtle – a GP might lose a large proportion of his patients and hence affect his income if he tries to impose a very different attitude concerning prescribing to that of his patients. One often has to move slowly in these matters.

For example, a study in London in the 1990s (Morgan, 1995) examined the attitudes of white and Afro-Caribbean patients with hypertension to their medicines and medicine taking. The white patients were more likely than the Afro-Caribbeans to take their medicines as prescribed, and tended to have better blood pressure control as a result. The Afro-Caribbean patients often had traditional cultural beliefs about long-term harmful effects of drugs and often sought an alternative resource in terms of herbal remedies. There was a cultural gulf and lack of communication between Afro-Caribbean patients and their GPs who did not appreciate these issues.

But even within what might seem to be a homogeneous culture, there can be wide variations in subcultures. For instance, within white British populations, attitudes to medicines will vary from the well heeled Sunday Times reader who wants to discuss a range of therapeutic options for a problem including complementary treatments, to many older more stoical patients who do not want to trouble the doctor, to other patients who want medicines (any medicines!) for every little ailment.

The key point is that one should not stereotype patients and that every patient is different, and deserves and needs to have their own needs and beliefs explored if the prescriber is to help the patient properly.

PATIENTS AND THE MEDIA

Increasingly the media influence us all in our day-to-day habits, in the food we eat, or the presents we purchase for Christmas and birthdays, and perhaps even in the medicines we swallow. The media portrays sensation and tends to see medicines either as 'wonder drugs' or as 'killer drugs': the notion that what is a wonder drug in one situation can also be a killer in another is a subtlety that banner headlines cannot deal with. In recent years, the media coverage for some new drugs has been intense, for instance of sildenafil (Viagra) – perhaps a potent mix of sex, money and science! This has certainly raised public awareness of the drug which may be good if it allows some patients with conditions which can be helped by sildenafil to overcome their reticence and come forward, but which may be harmful if encourages the use of this drug for normal men who feel that their sexual prowess could be enhanced further. There has been little in the media about the potential adverse medical effects of this drug. It is less clear what the actual effects of media coverage have been, in terms of encouraging drug sales. Nevertheless, newspapers and television can greatly increase awareness of a drug and its use when this has a very weak scientific basis.

Another example might be the uptake of vaccinations with measles/mumps/rubella (MMR), which has fallen drastically after adverse publicity that it might be associated with autism or inflammatory bowel disease. Statements by various scientific bodies have not been able to redress the powerful negative perceptions in some parts of the general public and as a result, there is now a real risk of an epidemic of these possibly serious childhood illnesses. While the scientific evidence is soundly in favour of immunisation, the public have had doubts instilled in their minds by the constant media hype, creating uncertainty. The positive images of the unbounded benefits of science of the1950s and 1960s has given way to a much more guarded view of science, largely as a result of many problems and disasters ranging from thalidomide to pollution. The social group most influenced against immunisation are the middle classes, perhaps reflecting better education in some areas (but not often in science).

In Europe, companies are not allowed to advertise their prescription-only-drugs to the general public, but are allowed advertise over the counter medicines generally. Despite this ban, there is a steady business in the media of almost 'advertorials' in newspapers and magazines that effectively promote particular prescription-only-drugs. In countries where direct advertising of prescription medicines is allowed, such as New Zealand or the US, there have been many concerns about the harmful effects of encouraging patients to seek perhaps inappropriate drugs. In the US, many drugs are openly advertised on the internet, where there is a plethora of information available – some good, some appallingly poor. This is all increasingly accessible to patients everywhere, so there may seem to be plenty of information available – in reality, such an information overload can often result in patients ending up more poorly informed about their drugs as a result of misinformation.

There is a dilemma here: the professionals might like the public's access to such information restricted since it might actually harm patients (but also might diminish their professional power): on the other hand, it might benefit patients who are not receiving medicines they should, or who can learn more about the medicines they are taking. The key concern here should be access to unbiased information, which we should encourage, but which is sadly not often available. Healthcare professionals have to help patients through this morass.

So the media can be a powerful influence with both advantages and disadvantages, and one that is likely to persist.

CONCLUSIONS

We have briefly examined a wide range of psychological and sociological influences on prescribing that act either directly on doctors or on patients (and hence indirectly on the doctors). There is little information or study so far of non-medical prescribers but it is very likely that all of the influences we have listed (and many we have not) will also affect nurses, pharmacists and others in the same way. They may be even more influential in the short-term in nurses and pharmacists, since dealing with these influences is part of medical culture handed down from trainer to trainee – this experience dose not exist yet with other professions. These issues will be of great importance in helping patients to use their medicines properly, and in achieving concordance with them about the aims and details of their treatment.

There are two key areas of skills to be learnt to remedy any potential harmful effect of these influences:

- *Self-reflection*: to be aware of these influences, and to recognise them when they occur; to be able to reflect on one's one prescribing and consider how influential these are on you as a prescriber; and to compare your prescribing and behaviour in this respect to that of your peers, or better still to some professional ideal. Then you can decide whether you have struck the proper balance.

● *Consultation*: where good communication (listening to the patient and understanding their point of view, as well as getting yours across to them) and an ability to negotiate (being prepared to trade, agree compromise and sell the deal) are essential.

References

Ivan Illich (1981). *Medical Nemesis*. London: Penguin.

Gilbert D, Walley T, New B (2000). Lifestyle medicines. *British Medical Journal* **321**: 1341–1344.

Harris CM, Heywood PL, Clayden AD (1990). *The Analysis of Prescribing in General Practice: A Guide to Audit and Research*. London: HMSO.

Howie JG (1976). Clinical judgement and antibiotic use in general practice. *British Medical Journal* **2**: 1061–1064.

Bradley CP (1991). Decision making and prescribing patterns – a literature review. *Family Practice* **8**: 276–287.

Anon (1983). Getting good value from drug reps. *Drugs and Therapeutics Bulletin* **21(4)**: 13–15.

Britten N, Ukoumunne OC, Boulton MG (2002). Patients' attitudes to medicines and expectations for prescriptions. *Health Expect* **5**: 256–269.

Macfarlane J, Holmes W, Macfarlane R, Britten N (1997). Influence of patients' expectations on antibiotic management of acute lower respiratory tract illness in general practice: questionnaire study. *British Medical Journal* **315**: 1211–1214.

Little P *et al.* (1997). Reattendance and complications in a randomised trial of prescribing strategies for sore throat: the medicalising effect of prescribing antibiotics. *British Medical Journal* **315**: 350–352.

Morgan M (1995). The significance of ethnicity for health promotion – patients use of antihypertensive drugs in inner London. *International Journal of Epidemiology* **24(suppl 1)**: S79–S84.

Chapter 7

Applied pharmacology

Michele Cossey

INTRODUCTION

Clinical pharmacology is defined as the application of scientific principles to understanding the ways in which drugs behave and work in humans (Weatherall, 2003).

A good general understanding of basic pharmacology and how it is applied to the treatment of patients is essential for any prescriber. It is not enough to have knowledge of how an individual drug may exert its effect. A prescriber must also understand how differences in individuals and populations may alter this effect. This understanding will allow prescribers to make decisions about route of administration, dosing, the frequency of administration, contraindications, adverse effects and interactions with other drugs. In order to be able to prescribe appropriately and effectively, prescribers need to appreciate the concepts of how the body handles drugs, i.e. *pharmacokinetics* and how these may be altered or influenced and, once in the body, how drugs can exert their effect and what may alter this potential effect, i.e. *pharmacodynamics*.

This chapter covers the essential elements of basic applied pharmacology. It will aim to give readers an overview of the general concepts of both pharmacokinetics and pharmacodynamics and how these influence drug choice, dose and effect. It will also look at adverse drug reactions (ADRs) and interactions, how these may occur and what the prescriber can do to minimise these where possible. Finally, it will bring the knowledge of these concepts together in order to provide a practical framework for individualising drug therapy.

In a chapter of this length, it is only possible to give a general overview. A more in-depth review of this subject can be found in McGavock (2003). Other further reading is provided at the end of this chapter.

PHARMACOKINETIC PRINCIPLES

Pharmacokinetics can simplistically be described as how the body handles drugs over a period of time. It is a complex subject but a general understanding of the basic principles is essential for good prescribing practice. The basic principles that a prescriber needs to have knowledge of are: absorption, distribution, metabolism and excretion (ADME) together with the route and dose of drug administered. The general principles of ADME can be summarised in Figure 7.1. These will be explained further in the following sections.

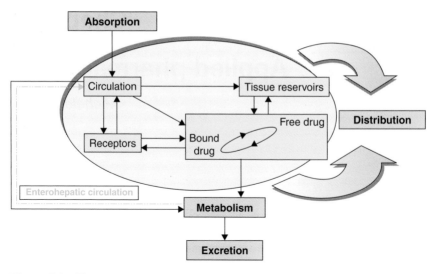

Figure 7.1   The general principles of ADME

ROUTES OF ADMINISTRATION

Drugs may act locally or systemically. Locally implies that the effects of the drug are confined to a specific area. Systemically means that a drug has to enter the circulation in order to be delivered to its site of action. Drugs may be administered to a patient in a number of different ways for example via the mouth (orally), via the skin (transdermally), via a mucous membrane (sublingual tablets) or via an injectable route (parenteral administration). The method of delivery into the body will influence the amount of drug reaching the circulation, intended site of action and ultimately, the effect of that drug. The term *bioavailability* is used to explain what proportion of an administered dose will reach the circulation unaltered, and therefore be able to have an effect. A drug given by intravenous (IV) injection will have a bioavailability of 1.0 as 100% of the dose is administered directly into the circulation. A drug given by the oral route will have a reduced bioavailability due to the effects of ADME. The chosen route of administration will depend on many factors including, condition to be treated, the speed of required drug action, patient preference and available methods of delivery. The prescriber's main aim is to select the most appropriate route of administration that will be both clinically useful and cost-effective. For example, in the treatment of asthma, drug therapy is delivered by inhaler directly into the lungs where the effect is required, whilst in the case of eczema, drug therapy may be applied directly to the affected area. What the prescriber must do is make an initial decision based on the absorption of the drug into the body and the required site of action.

ABSORPTION

The process of absorption brings the drug from its site of action into the body's general circulation. Almost all drugs, other than those for example administered by IV injection must be absorbed before they can exert their effect. Drugs that exert their effect systemically must cross at least one cell in order to reach the circulation. Most drugs do this by passive diffusion (i.e. movement from an area of high concentration to an area of low concentration) for example, in crossing through the wall of the small intestine, where there is high concentration, into the blood stream, where there is low concentration. However, some drugs (e.g. levadopa and fluorouracil) will require special transport mechanisms in order to cross cell membranes. These 'active transport' mechanisms are not very important for the absorption of other drugs but are essential in ensuring maintenance of cellular function by transport of ions for example potassium (K^+), sugars and amino acids across cell walls.

The rate and extent of drug absorption across a cell membrane will be determined by a number of factors.

Lipid solubility

The lipid solubility of a drug will determine how easily it will pass across a cell membrane. Cell membranes are composed of a double layer of phospholipids and so lipid soluble drugs (or lipophilic drugs) will pass though cell membranes more easily than water-soluble drugs. Another determination is the state of ionisation of a drug, as only un-ionised drug is lipid soluble. Therefore, the more lipid soluble a drug, the easier it is for that drug to be absorbed from the small intestine after oral administration. This fact is used in the design and manufacture of drugs. For example, if a manufacturer wanted to formulate a drug to act directly within the gut for example for Crohn's disease, they would look to develop a water-soluble (or low lipid-soluble) drug, so that the drug is held within the gut and not absorbed from the small intestine.

Surface area for absorption

The larger the surface area available for absorption, the quicker the process will occur. The small intestine has a very large surface area for drug absorption to take place, due to a large number of villi and a very rich blood supply. If a patient has a condition that reduces the potential area for drug absorption for example inflammatory bowel disease, then the relative absorption of a drug will be reduced, thus interfering with the amount of drug available in the circulation and ultimately, the effect of that drug.

Gastric motility and emptying

Most absorption takes place in the small intestine. This means that drugs taken orally need to be disintegrated in the stomach and delivered via emptying of the gastric contents into the intestine. Therefore, anything that alters gastric motility and emptying will result in altering the rate of absorption.

The presence of food after a meal will slow gastric emptying. If drugs are taken with food, then their absorption and effect may be delayed. This is why it is important to ensure that drugs are prescribed to be taken either before or some time after a meal. This ensures quicker delivery to the site of absorption and prevents delaying the drug effect. This is why counselling the patient on when to take their drugs is very important. Sometimes drugs are prescribed 'to be taken with food'. This is to lessen side-effects by preventing large concentrations from entering the circulation so that the drug is absorbed in a steadier manner, due to slower gastric emptying. It is also to prevent local side-effects, like irritation of the stomach lining by using the food as a barrier.

Some illnesses or conditions may affect this process. Gastric emptying may be slowed during a migraine attack and therefore, oral analgesics may not act quickly enough. This can be addressed by giving the drug via another route for example subcutaneous injection or by combining the oral analgesic with a drug to speed up gastric motility for example metoclopramide.

However, the whole process of gastric motility and emptying and its effect on drug absorption is very complex. In some cases, delayed gastric emptying may actually be beneficial to drug absorption. For example, some drugs, such as nitrofurantoin, may be better dissolved or disintegrated as a result of spending longer in the stomach's acidic environment.

First pass metabolism

Some drugs when given orally are absorbed from the small intestine directly into the hepatic portal vein and to the liver. As the liver is the main organ for metabolism, these drugs are then metabolised either partially or fully by the liver. This means that the amount of drug entering the circulation is either reduced or completely negated. This effect is known as *first pass metabolism*. Some drugs for example glyceryl trinitrate, when swallowed are almost totally inactivated via the first pass metabolism effect and are therefore administered by another route. In the case of glyceryl trinitrate, by sublingual spray or injection. Other drugs may still be active even after first pass metabolism if their metabolites are active for example propranolol metabolised to the active 4-hydroxypropranolol. This is why it is important to understand the bioavailability of a drug. In practical terms, prescribers can often assume that a drug has been formulated to take account of any first past metabolism effect and therefore, rarely have to consider it.

Time

The amount of time that a drug is in contact with the walls of the small intestine will affect its absorption. Anything that alters gut transit time for example, gastroenteritis will affect time for absorption. Conversely, hypomotility of the gastrointestinal tract may result in higher concentrations of drug entering the circulation.

Blood flow

Depending on how drugs are administered, the blood flow to the site of administration will affect the rate of absorption. Blood flow to the gut is usually high and this allows for good absorption into the circulation. Some areas of the body have variable blood flow for example muscles and so absorption from intramuscular injection may vary, depending on other physical aspects of the patient which may require muscle blood flow to be increased or decreased.

As described above, there are a number of factors that will influence the absorption of a drug from its site of action into the circulation. Sometimes, a drug may not be given by what seems the most obvious route for example choosing a matrix skin patch in chronic pain relief, rather than an oral formulation. Unless a prescriber understands how these factors affect drug absorption, they will not be able to pick the appropriate formulation and route of administration to ensure effective absorption and delivery of the drug to its site of action.

DISTRIBUTION

Once a drug is absorbed from its site of administration into the circulation it is transported around the body to its site of action. This process is known as distribution. Unless a drug reaches its site of action in an adequate concentration, it will not be able to exert its effect. As with absorption, there are factors that will influence the distribution of drugs around the body.

Blood flow

The rate and extent to which organs and tissues are perfused with blood will directly affect the distribution of drug to those areas. This, in turn, will affect the rate and extent of drug action at that site. Organs and tissues that receive high blood perfusion for example heart, kidneys and brain will rapidly receive a drug and have a much greater potential of receiving an adequate concentration for the drug to have an effect. Poorly perfused organs and tissues for example fat, muscle and bone may take some time to receive adequate drug concentrations.

Protein binding

Most drugs that enter the circulation are poorly soluble. This means that in order to move around the body via the circulatory system, some proportion of the drug needs to be 'carried'. These 'carriers' are plasma proteins and drug molecules are either 'free' in the circulation or 'bound' to these proteins. It should be noted that only free drug can cross plasma membranes and therefore can exert an effect (as drugs bound to plasma proteins are large). This state of plasma binding is a reversible process. A drug may enter the circulation and be partially or wholly bound to plasma proteins but overtime the drug is released from this protein binding site or free drug may bind to plasma proteins. This is a dynamic process that allows for equilibrium to be reached between the fraction of bound and unbound (free) drug.

Albumin is the most abundant plasma protein and generally, drugs that are acidic in nature bind to albumin, whilst drugs that are alkali in nature bind to α_1-acid glycoprotein. The process of drug binding to plasma protein is a competitive one. This means that if more than one drug that binds to plasma protein is present at the same time in the circulation, these drugs will compete for the plasma protein binding sites.

This is an important concept to understand, particularly for drugs that are highly protein-bound and have a *narrow therapeutic index* (e.g. warfarin). A narrow therapeutic index means that the concentration of drug needed to have an effect is

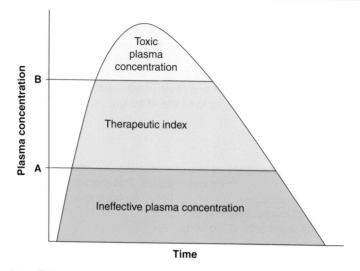

Figure 7.2   Diagrammatic representation of therapeutic index

very close to that which may be either toxic or ineffective. This is shown in Figure 7.2. If warfarin is competing with other drugs for binding sites, more of it may be displaced from these binding sites and will therefore be free in the circulation. This free drug will then be metabolised and excreted. However, if there are any problems with excretion or metabolism, for example poor renal or liver function then the effect of this free warfarin can be problematic as it may cause the patient to bleed due to higher free plasma concentration exerting a potentially greater effect. Tolbutamide is an example of a drug which competes with, and can displace warfarin from, its binding sites.

Interactions of this type are more likely to be clinically important in the acute setting for example in administering loading doses of warfarin before steady state is reached. Once a drug has reached steady state then small amounts being displaced from protein binding sites will have less significant effects as metabolism and excretion will deal with these. This is one of the reasons why patients taking warfarin have their International Normalised Ratio (INR), a measure of the blood's clotting time checked regularly and this monitoring is increased when they are started on other drugs known to interact with warfarin, until they are stabilised on the new combination.

This situation could also theoretically arise if a patient is suffering from a disease that alters plasma proteins. In a patient with for example a chronic liver disease (e.g. cirrhosis), drug dosing can be altered to take account of lower albumin concentrations. However, if a patient stabilised on warfarin suddenly develops an acute liver problem, which leads to altered albumin production then drugs that would routinely be bound to albumin may be free in the circulation in higher concentrations than expected and exert a greater than anticipated effect. Figure 7.3 shows the potential impact of altered protein binding on plasma drug concentration.

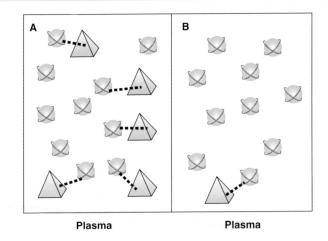

Plasma   **Plasma**

In **A** there is an equilibrium between free drug and drug-bound to plasma proteins

In **B** as the concentration of the plasma protein falls (for example in liver disease) the concentration of free drug X increases.

As free drug is active there is more drug available to target receptors and have an increased effect.

Figure 7.3 The potential impact of altered protein binding on plasma drug concentration

For the prescriber, it is important to understand this concept of protein binding in order to make a decision about drug dosing. In patients with reduced hepatic function or disease states that may impact on plasma protein concentrations, drug doses of highly protein-bound drugs should be reduced.

Distribution barriers

For a drug to have an effect, it must reach the tissues. Drugs can access and accumulate in certain tissues or cannot gain access to other tissues, due to the existence of barriers. The blood–brain barrier is made up of different endothelial cells that only allow highly lipid soluble drugs to cross over into the brain tissue. A drug that is poorly lipid soluble will have great difficulty in crossing this barrier and will have little or no effect on the brain. However, an anaesthetic agent, which is formulated to be highly lipid soluble, will pass through this barrier. Whilst some of the anaesthetic may pass into other tissues (e.g. muscle or fat stores) the vast majority of the drug will cross the blood–brain barrier and as the brain has a higher blood perfusion than that of muscle or fat, the drug will have the desired effect of rapid anaesthesia.

In pregnancy, the placenta forms a barrier between the mother's circulation and that of the fetus. Some drugs which are highly lipophilic can cross this barrier, for example morphine, ethanol, whilst other poorly lipid-soluble molecules cannot easily pass through.

Volume of distribution

When a drug is given and enters the circulation, it may bind to plasma proteins (as described above) in order to be carried around the body. Once in the general circulation, the drug can exert its effect by binding to specific receptor sites or it may bind to other tissues where it has no pharmacological effect, for example fat stores or certain organs. The term *volume of distribution* can describe the extent to which a drug is distributed throughout the body and bound to other tissues. Those drugs that are highly distributed throughout body tissues may have a lower plasma concentration and therefore, a higher dose may be required compared to a drug that undergoes little tissue distribution and the majority of which stays within the circulation.

In practical terms, the prescriber can assume that the volume of distribution of a drug has been taken into account during the formulation of that drug. However, an understanding of this concept may be useful in drug overdose where for example, haemodialysis is used to try and clear the drug from the circulation. If most of the drug is distributed and bound to other tissues, i.e. the volume of distribution is high and little of the drug is actually present in the circulation, then haemodialysis may be ineffective.

A more in-depth view of the volume of distribution can be found in some of the further reading at the end of this chapter.

Once a drug is in the circulation and distributed around the body, in order to have its effect, the body must have mechanisms in place to excrete the drug. In order to effectively excrete drugs from the body, they are first metabolised.

METABOLISM

Drug metabolism or biotransformation is the process of modifying or altering the chemical composition of the drug. As described previously, the more lipid soluble and un-ionised a drug, the more easily it passes across cell membranes. It would seem logical then, that in order to remove the pharmacological activity and actively excrete a drug, the body should attempt to make the drug more water soluble (hydrophilic) and less lipid soluble, as well as making the drug more polar (or ionised). This means that when a drug enters the kidney for excretion, it is unlikely to be reabsorbed across the cell membranes back into the general circulation.

Most drug metabolism occurs in the liver where a series of enzymes catalyse numerous biochemical reactions. These reactions can be classified into two phases: *Phase 1 and Phase 2*. Some drugs may undergo both Phase 1 and Phase 2 metabolism, some may undergo only one of these phases and some may undergo Phase 2 before Phase 1. There are also some drugs that are excreted unchanged, without being actively metabolised.

Phase 1

The process of Phase 1 metabolism results in oxidation, reduction or hydrolysis of a drug. The process of oxidation is the most common and often catalysed by one of the many Cytochrome P450 isoenzymes (CYP450). Although the aim of this process is to render the drug less effective and more water soluble, some drugs are actually made pharmacologically active by this process, for example enalapril is pharmacologically inactive, but its Phase 1 metabolite enalaprilat is active. In some cases, the resulting metabolite of an active drug is itself pharmacologically active (e.g. diamorphine metabolised to morphine).

Phase 2

Drugs or phase 1 metabolites that are not sufficiently polar, or are still active, are made more hydrophilic by the process of conjugation. This process involves the drug or metabolite being attached to an endogenous compound, for example, a glucuronate. The resulting compounds are more readily excreted by the kidneys, as they are more water soluble and polar in nature. As with Phase 1, some drugs are still active after conjugation (e.g. morphine is metabolised to morphine-6-glucuronide), which still exerts analgesic effect.

Cytochrome P450 iso-enzymes

Before leaving drug metabolism, it is necessary to take a closer look at the CYP450 enzyme group and how affecting these enzymes can have major effects on the excretion of certain drugs.

Some drugs can increase the rate of synthesis and action of CYP450 enzymes and are known as enzyme inducers (e.g. rifampicin), whilst other drugs can inhibit this process and are known as drug inhibitors (e.g. cimetidine). (Table 7.1 gives some examples of clinically important inducers and inhibitors.) Generally, induction requires that the CYP450 enzymes are exposed to the enzyme inducer for some time, whilst enzyme inhibitors can exert their effect on the CYP450 system soon after exposure.

Sometimes, it is not just drugs that can affect this CYP450 system. Exogenous substances can also affect it and if these substances are taken at the same time as drug therapy, then they can affect the action of the drug. A good example of

Table 7.1   Examples of CYP450 enzyme inducers and inhibitors

CYP450 Inhibitors	CYP450 Inducers
Amiodarone	Carbamazepine
Cimetidine	Phenytoin
Ciprofloxacin	Rifampicin
Erythromycin	Alcohol
Metronidazole	
Omperazole	

NB. Not a complete list. Prescribers should always check appropriate texts if in doubt.

this is grapefruit juice, which is known to induce the CYP450 system. Patients taking drugs where plasma concentration is crucial, due to a narrow therapeutic index e.g. theophylline or cyclosporin, are advised not to drink grapefruit juice, as it can result in speeding up the enzyme system and result in a much reduced plasma concentration and therapeutic effect of the drug. A full list of enzyme inducers and inhibitors can be found in the British National Formulary (BNF).

Most drugs are metabolised by concentration-independent mechanisms, i.e. the enzyme responsible for their metabolism is not saturated, whilst the drug is within the therapeutic range. There are some enzymes that can be saturated even when the drug is within this therapeutic range. As this happens, small additional doses can lead to a disproportionate rise in plasma concentration and ultimately, to toxicity. An example of this is the drug phenytoin (an antiepileptic). This drug has a narrow therapeutic index and the enzyme responsible for its metabolism becomes saturated within its therapeutic range, so small increases in dose can cause increases in plasma concentrations above the therapeutic level and result in toxicity. As there is great inter-patient variability in this response, phenytoin requires careful dosing and plasma monitoring, until a patient is stable.

As discussed the processes of drug metabolism are aimed at making a drug more readily excreted.

EXCRETION

Most drugs are excreted via the kidney either unchanged or after the processes of metabolism. As described above, the process of drug metabolism may result in a pharmacologically active compound and therefore, the effect of the drug will mainly be dependant on excretion, rather than its metabolism.

Renal excretion

The kidneys are very well perfused, receiving approximately 1.5 l per minute of blood. A proportion of this (between 10% and 20%) is actively filtered by the glomerulus producing glomelular filtrate. Some drugs or metabolites can pass directly into the kidney at this stage, but they have to be small and therefore, drugs or metabolites bound to plasma proteins cannot pass into the kidney in this way, but unbound or free drugs can.

Some drugs are actively secreted from the capillaries into the proximal convoluted tubule of the nephron. This process of tubular secretion is an active process requiring carrier systems and, usually, involves those drugs or metabolites that are strongly acidic or alkali in nature. An example of a drug excreted in this way is penicillin. As this process is an active one, it can be inhibited by, for example, the drug probenecid, which inhibits the active transport mechanism and therefore, the excretion of penicillin, thereby increasing the plasma concentration of penicillin.

Some drugs are actively reabsorbed back into the circulation. Active reabsorption enables the body to hold onto vital nutrients and vitamins. Drugs which are still lipid soluble and un-ionised at urine pH can be reabsorbed during this process and continue to exert their effect. Excretion of these drugs can be influenced by altering the pH of urine, e.g. by administering sodium bicarbonate.

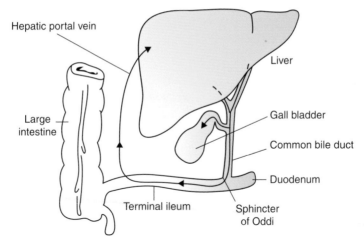

Figure 7.4 The enterohepatic circulation

Enterohepatic cycling

Other mechanisms of drug excretion include via the liver, in bile. Once secreted by the liver into bile, they enter the duodenum via the common bile duct and continue on towards the small intestine. Here, some drugs can be deconjugated by the action of gut bacteria and reabsorbed back into the blood stream from the terminal ileum. They then return to the liver by the enterohepatic circulation. The drug undergoes further metabolism and is secreted back into bile and continues going around this process called *enterohepatic cycling*. Figure 7.4 shows this process.

This is an important mechanism to understand because although not many drugs are excreted in bile, those that are and that undergo this cycling mechanism, can have their effect in the body extended but also, anything that interferes with this mechanism, can alter the effect of the drug. For example, the oral contraceptive pill contains oestrogens that are recycled around the body by this mechanism. If a woman is given a course of broad-spectrum antibiotics, these could alter the gut bacteria and therefore, metabolites are not broken down in the small intestine. The oestrogen conjugate is excreted in faeces and enterohepatic cycling is prevented. This can reduce the effect of the oral contraceptive pill. Similarly, diarrhoea can limit the time available for this cycling and also reduce the effect of the pill.

Other methods of excretion

Other methods of excretion include via sweat, breath, tears, saliva and breast milk. These are passive processes and tend to be less important except, of course, when prescribing for nursing mothers. A list of drugs that are excreted in breast milk is available in the BNF.

Half-life

The term *half-life* ($t_{1/2}$) of a drug is used to describe the time it takes for the plasma concentration to fall to half its original value and is measured in hours. Figure 7.5

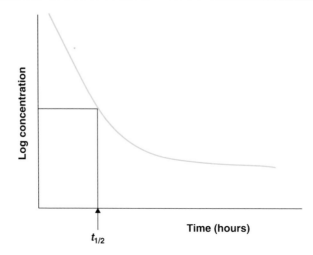

Figure 7.5   Graphical illustration of half-life ($t_{1/2}$)

shows this graphically. This is an important factor, as those drugs with very short half-lives (rapidly excreted) will have to be administered very frequently, to ensure adequate plasma concentrations compared to those with longer half-lives, which can be administered at greater intervals.

When a drug is given in repeated doses, there will come a point when the drug begins to accumulate and a state arises where elimination of the drug by the body matches that being given by the administered dose. This is termed *'steady state'*. Drugs with short half-lives reach steady state quicker than those with long half-lives. In order to reach steady state with a drug that has a long half-life, a loading dose may be needed to achieve a therapeutic plasma concentration and this is then followed by smaller maintenance doses, to maintain this plasma concentration or steady state.

Having dealt with the key principles of ADME, the prescriber can use this under-standing to make some assessments of drug dosing. By using the information already described in this chapter, a prescriber should be able to consider the follow-ing points. When a drug is administered, the route of administration determines how quickly it will have its effect. The amount of drug in the circulation and its potential effect will depend on how much is administered, whether the drug is plasma protein bound or free (i.e. how it distributed around the body), receptor binding properties (see later section) and how quickly it is metabolised and excreted. The speed at which a drug is treated by the body is one of the key factors in determining the duration of action of that drug. These are the principles of pharmacokinetics.

PHARMACODYNAMICS

In the first section, we dealt with how the body deals with drugs, or pharmaco-kinetics. Pharmacodynamics studies the effects that the drug will have on the body, at both receptor level and on the body's systems as a whole.

The many and varied physiological systems and mechanisms that control all bodily functions are very complex. These functions are kept in check by a myriad of

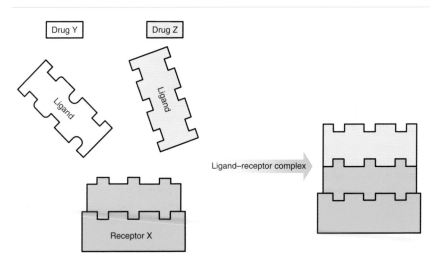

Figure 7.6   Drug–receptor binding. Drug Y cannot bind to Receptor X as it is the wrong shape whereas drug Z has a complementary structure and can therefore bind to Receptor X to form a ligand–receptor complex

different electrical and chemical messenger systems that work together to maintain the body's homoeostatic state. There are many different ways in which the body controls its systems by signalling from one to another in order to switch systems on, off or alter their rate. The body's own endogenous signals that act on receptors are often called *ligands*. The body could not function as it does without the presence of these natural ligands. For example insulin, noradrenalin and serotonin are all naturally occurring chemical substances within the body that exert their effects by acting as ligands at receptor sites. The body's many types of signalling are too varied and complex to review in detail in this chapter but in-depth reviews of this subject can be found in the further reading at the end of the chapter.

Drugs exert their effect by altering to a lesser or greater degree the body's own physiological systems. In this way drugs act as exogenous ligands. Drugs can act at receptors, at enzyme systems, at ion channels or at carrier mechanisms.

DRUGS ACTING AT RECEPTORS

Drugs have their effect at receptors by mimicking an endogenous (natural) ligand and binding to a receptor site in the same manner that one of the body's own signalling molecules might do, to form a *ligand–receptor complex*. The receptor sites are usually protein molecules either on the surface of a cell or located intracellularly in the cytoplasm. Obviously drugs act in many different ways and this is because not all drugs can bind to all receptors. In order for a drug to act as a ligand at a particular receptor site it must have a complementary structure to that site. This can be considered in the same way as jigsaw pieces fitting together (Figure 7.6).

As discussed above, drugs bind to receptor sites. However, not all drugs bind to their chosen receptors to the same degree. The term *affinity* is used to describe the extent to which a drug binds to a receptor. The greater affinity a drug has for a receptor the greater the binding between the drug and its chosen receptor will be. Some drugs have greater or lesser affinity for their receptors than others.

Whilst drugs may exert an effect at a receptor, the extent and type of this effect will also vary. The effect of the ligand–receptor complex will vary depending on how the drug exerts its effect. In some cases this drug–ligand complex causes a specific response and these types of ligands are called *agonists*. An example of a drug acting as an agonist is salbutamol, a beta$_2$–receptor agonist used in asthma, which binds to receptors on the smooth muscle in the bronchioles causing bronchodilation. Some ligand–drug complexes do not have an effect but they stop or block a particular natural messenger system from having its effect and this type of ligand is called an *antagonist*. An example of a drug acting as an antagonist is atenolol, a beta$_1$-adrenoceptor antagonist used in angina. It is used to block the β_1 effects of adrenaline on the heart, causing a slowing of the force of contraction, reduction in cardiac oxygen consumption and alleviation of angina pain.

DRUG DOSE – RESPONSE, AGONISTS AND ANTAGONISTS

Drugs are given to exert a desired effect. Each drug will have a maximum attainable response, which is dependant on the concentration of the drug in the body. The maximum drug response is termed E_{max} and the concentration of drug required to exert half its maximum effect is termed EC_{50}. This is shown in Figure 7.7.

Agonists can be described as either *complete or partial agonists.* A drug is a complete agonist if it can exert its maximal effect when all receptors are occupied. If it can only exert a sub-maximal effect (i.e. less than the body's own natural agonist effect) when all receptors are occupied, it is termed a partial agonist. The term *efficacy* is used to describe the ability of a drug to exert an effect at a receptor site. We can say that agonists have both affinity for, and efficacy at, receptor sites but whilst antagonists have affinity for receptor sites, they do not directly exert an effect and so have no efficacy. As described above drugs have to be present in certain concentrations in the body in order to exert their effects. The term *potency*

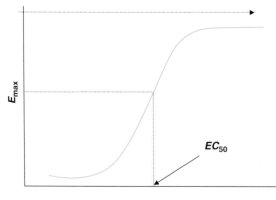

Log concentration

Figure 7.7   Dose–response curve

is used to describe the relative concentration (or dose) of a drug that has to be present in order to produce the desired effect. The more potent a drug, the less that has to be administered for a given effect. These concepts can be shown in Figure 7.8 where the drug response (effect) is plotted against log concentration for drugs of varying agonist effect, efficacy and potency.

As described above, antagonists stop or block a system by occupying a receptor site. The body will still be producing its own natural chemical messengers (ligands) but these cannot exert their usual effect at a receptor site in the presence of the antagonist. Antagonists can be *competitive or non-competitive* in nature. A competitive antagonist will compete with the natural ligand for receptor sites and form a reversible bond. As more drug antagonist is made available (e.g. by giving further doses and increasing the concentration of drug in the body's circulation) then the antagonist is able to occupy more receptors than the agonist and more of the body's own natural response is blocked. In order to overcome this effect more of the body's own natural agonist needs to be made available in order to compete with the antagonist for these receptor sites, i.e. competition needs to be set up between agonist and antagonist. A non-competitive antagonist also forms a bond at a receptor site but often this bond is almost irreversible. Therefore, no matter how much of the natural agonist is present, the antagonist still exerts its effect.

Drugs acting at enzyme systems

Some drugs have their effect by altering the effect of the body's enzyme systems. Sometimes, the drug may resemble the enzyme's natural substrate and so

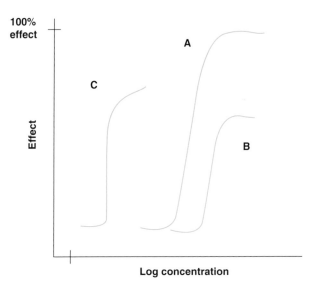

Figure 7.8   Agonists, efficacy and potency. Drug A is a full agonist as it exerts maximal effect when all receptors are occupied whilst drug B is only a partial agonist. Drug A and B are equipotent but A is more efficacious. Drug C is more potent than A or B.

competition is set up between the drug and the natural substrate for binding to the enzyme. Other times, the drug may bind irreversibly to the enzyme's active site, therefore rendering it unable to carry out its usual function. An example of a drug acting on an enzyme system is that of the angiotensin converting enzyme inhibitors (ACEIs) which block the enzymatic conversion by renin of the physiologically inactive angiotensin I to the vasoconstrictor angiotensin II. These ACEIs are used to control blood pressure by preventing vasoconstriction as well as having other indications.

Drugs acting at ion channels

Sometimes in the body a system is controlled by cells allowing the selective movement of certain ions across cell membranes, for example calcium (Ca^{2+}) or potassium (K^+) ions, which sets up an electrical potential gradient across the membrane. Anything that alters this selective movement across a cell membrane can alter this electrical potential and therefore, affect that body system. For example, calcium channel blocker drugs (e.g. nifedipine, diltiazem) act by blocking natural channels across cell membranes, which under certain situations allow the passage of calcium ions across smooth muscle cells. This results in an altered electrical potential and therefore an altered physiological response in this case a reduced force of contraction of smooth muscle in the heart.

Drugs acting on carrier mechanisms

In the first section of this chapter we discussed the process of active transport systems that allowed certain ions and molecules to be maintained at different concentrations in different cells of the body. These active transport systems are energy dependant carrier mechanisms and some drugs can interfere with these mechanisms. Examples include digoxin which blocks the H^+/K^+ pump in the heart and the proton pump inhibitor drugs like omeprazole, which block the Na^+/K^+ pump in the gastric mucosa.

Further in-depth discussions of the concepts described in this section can be found in the further reading at the end of this chapter.

As we can see the concepts of **pharmacokinetics** and **pharmacodynamics** are very complex. It is important that prescribers have at least a basic understanding of these, in order to be able to predict and individualise drug therapy. They are also important in understanding how drugs interact and why drugs can exert unwanted or adverse effects.

DRUG INTERACTIONS

It is not difficult to understand that just as the body's own systems do not work in isolation, but interact to maintain a homoeostatic environment, that when two or more drugs are administered to a patient, there is the potential for these drugs to interact with each other. Although pharmacologically two or more drugs may interact, the interaction may not always lead to a clinically significant effect. Drug interactions that are clinically significant can be harmful or sometimes beneficial and may not occur in every patient.

It is not possible for prescribers to be aware of every potential drug interaction. By understanding how drugs can interact, in whom these interactions are more likely to occur and which drugs are most likely to be involved, they can apply this knowledge to their prescribing practice. If in doubt, prescribers should always check the literature or seek specialist advice before prescribing multiple drugs for patients.

Who is at risk of drug interactions?

Any patient receiving two or more drugs is at potential risk of a drug interaction. However, the greater the number of drugs a patient receives the greater the number of potential drug interactions. There are also some groups or individuals who may be more susceptible to drug interactions. These include:

The elderly
The elderly population generally receive a number of different drugs for the treatment of multiple conditions or to reduce the potential risk of future morbidities. Coupled with this fact, they may also have declining physiological functions, for example renal function may be impaired to some degree. For these reasons *polypharmacy* (the prescribing of a number of different drugs to one individual) increases the potential for drug interactions in this group of patients.

Seriously ill patients
Patients who are seriously ill or who have undergone a serious intervention for example organ transplant may be receiving numerous drugs and may have altered physiological functions as a result of their illness or condition.

Those who receive prescriptions from more than one prescriber
These days, a patient may have a prescription from their general practitioner (GP), their health visitor and a consultant and this is not an exhaustive list. As more healthcare professionals are given prescribing rights, the greater the risks for communication breakdown. Unless there are good communication channels between all prescribers and clear records are maintained, there is the potential for drug interactions to occur, due to lack of information being available at the time of prescribing.

Other groups
Other patient groups who are at potential risk include those taking drugs with a narrow therapeutic index (see section one), those with renal or hepatic impairment, patients taking over-the-counter medication, which is not documented in their records and those who require long-term drug therapies for a specific disease or condition.

Which drugs are more likely to be involved in drug interactions?

Whilst theoretically, any two drugs could interact, not all do and even if they do, the outcome may not be clinically significant. There are some drugs, which for a number of reasons are more likely to be involved in a drug interaction. These include drugs with a narrow therapeutic index, those that act on the CYP450 enzyme system, drugs that require the same protein carrier type, drugs that can act on the same receptor type. A list of drug interactions is given in the BNF and a prescriber must decide which could be clinically significant in their specific patient.

How do drugs interact?

There are many ways in which drugs can interact with one another. In this section, we will only consider drug interactions that occur in the body and not those which can occur before the drug is administered to a patient, due to, for example storage conditions. In describing how drugs can interact, we will refer to concepts and processes described in sections one and two of this chapter.

PHARMACOKINETIC DRUG INTERACTIONS

Drug interactions may occur at any stage of ADME. Regardless of which stage the interaction takes place, the overall effect is to alter the concentration of drug in the plasma and therefore, either increase or decrease its effect.

Absorption

Anything that interferes with the absorption of a drug from its site of administration will alter the bioavailability of the drug and ultimately, its effect. The most common type of drug interaction due to alteration of absorption occurs in the gastrointestinal tract. Some drugs may bind to another if given at the same time and so prevent the absorption of one of the drugs: for example antacids may reduce the absorption of some commonly used antibiotics. Hence the warnings that are put onto medicine bottles to avoid taking antacids at the same time as antibiotics. Other drugs may slow gastric emptying and so prolong the time it takes for another drug, given at the same time, to exert its effect. In other situations, giving a drug that increases gastric motility e.g. metoclopramide, may adversely affect the absorption of a drug that requires gastric acid to breakdown its outer layer, in order to activate the drug. For example, some enteric-coated drugs require a certain length of exposure to the acid environment of the stomach, in order to release the active drug. In section two of this chapter, the concept of enterohepatic circulation was discussed, in relation to the oral contraceptives and the interaction between this reabsorption process and antibiotics was also described.

Distribution

In section one, the factors that effect drug distribution were described and it was noted that only free drug is pharmacologically active. Drugs bound to plasma proteins are inactive. Some drugs are very heavily protein bound and if they are given at the same time as another highly protein bound drug, competition will exist between the two drugs for the same protein binding sites. This may mean that the concentration of either drug as 'free' drug may be increased or decreased, depending on which drug binds to the most protein binding sites. This may have no clinically significant effect but in certain situations, the effect could be very significant. An example of this type was discussed in section two under the heading of protein binding where the interaction of warfarin and tolbutamide was described in relation to concentrations of circulating proteins.

Metabolism

In section two, the CYP450 enzyme system was described. The fact that certain drugs could induce or inhibit this system was discussed, with examples. If a patient is stabilised on a drug (e.g. phenytoin) and then an enzyme inhibiting drug is given to that patient (e.g. erythromycin) then the metabolism of the phenytoin may be reduced (due to erythromycin, inhibiting the enzymes needed to metabolise phenytoin) leading to higher concentrations circulating in the body. As phenytoin is another drug with a narrow therapeutic index, small changes in its plasma concentrations can cause toxicity, as in this case, or reduction in effect. Prescribers should always consult the BNF for clinically important enzyme inducers or inhibitors and their potential drug interactions.

Excretion

Some drugs can alter the excretion of other drugs. For example, non-steroidal anti-inflammatory drugs (NSAIDs) like ibuprofen or diclofenac can reduce the renal excretion of lithium. Again lithium is a drug with a narrow therapeutic index, so reducing its excretion can have serious toxic side-effects.

PHARMACODYNAMIC DRUG INTERACTIONS

These can sometimes be predicted by knowing the mechanism of action of the drugs involved. There are too many to describe in this chapter but some common examples are described below.

Asthmatic patients are advised to avoid β-blocker drugs. This is because beta-receptors are present in the bronchioles and in the heart. So, in this example, an asthmatic patient relies on the agonist effect of salbutamol on β_2-receptors in the bronchioles to keep their airways open. If a β-blocker is given to this patient, there is the potential that it may block not only β_1-receptors in the heart, but also some β_2-receptors in the bronchioles. If this happens, it will antagonise the effect of the salbutamol and the patient may experience wheezing, or worse, the effect may precipitate an asthma attack due to reduced effect of the salbutamol. Although drugs are formulated to be more *selective* for one type of receptor than another e.g. β_1-selective β-blockers are formulated so that they act on the β_1-receptors in the heart but not those β_2-receptors in the bronchioles and smooth muscle, there is always the possibility that selectivity is not 100%, i.e. *selectivity* is relative.

ACEIs and NSAIDs can interact due to the effect that both increase fluid and K^+ concentrations. Digoxin used in controlling atrial fibrillation is affected by K^+ concentrations, so K^+ sparing diuretics e.g. amiloride can interact with digoxin.

Prescribers should always consult the BNF for clinically important drug-drug interactions, before prescribing for any patient taking more than one drug.

ADVERSE DRUG REACTIONS

Any drug given to a patient can cause an unintended harmful effect. This effect can be described as an 'Adverse Drug Reaction' (ADR). ADRs are very common and are thought to occur in between 10% and 20% of all patients prescribed drugs. ADRs are thought to be implicated in approximately 4% of all hospital admissions and are the cause of up to 10% of all GP consultations. One UK based study concluded that over a 9-week-study period of the 840 screened admissions to an adult acute ward, 85 (10.1%) were drug related and 52% of these were caused by an ADR (Bhalla *et al.*, 2003).

The problem with ADRs is that they may not be recognised as such but instead, considered to be an integral part of the patients' disease progression. As with drug interactions, it is not possible for a prescriber to have knowledge of all possible ADRs (particularly as some are idiosyncratic in nature). Prescribers should be vigilant and consider ADRs as one of the possible options when patients experience problems.

What are adverse drug reactions?

The classification of ADRs can be very complex and can be explored in more depth in the further reading suggested at the end of this chapter.

ADRs can be classified into two types: *Type A* and *Type B.*

Type A reactions
These are often predictable from the drug's pharmacology and are caused by an excessive or inadequate response to a drug. These can be the result of pharmacokinetic or pharmacodynamic problems. This type of ADR is often predictable; dose related, and can be managed, often by simple dose alteration. In fact, side-effects of drugs are Type A ADRs, an unwanted but predictable response to a drug. Some examples of Type A reactions include aminoglycoside (e.g. gentamicin) hearing impairment due to drug accumulation in patients with poor or impaired renal function, NSAID related peptic ulcer, due to the blockade of prostaglandin synthesis, which protect the stomach lining.

Type B reactions
These are idiosyncratic in nature, not predictable from the drug's pharmacology and therefore, unrelated to the dose of the drug. Although they are not as common as Type A reactions, they are clinically very important, as the effect of a Type B ADR can be very serious. An example would be an anaphylactic reaction to a therapeutic dose of penicillin.

Who is at risk of adverse drug reactions?

As discussed above, some ADRs are completely idiosyncratic and cannot be predicted. However, prescribers should be extra cautious in certain patient groups, including the elderly and the very young, (due to altered pharmacokinetic and pharmacodynamic processes), patients with renal or liver impairment or disease, patients with a known genetic predisposition e.g. glucose 6-phosphate dehydrogenase deficiency, who can suffer haemolysis when given certain drugs.

Reporting adverse drug reactions

Many rare Type B ADRs will not show up in pre-marketing drug testing, as not enough patients are exposed to the drug. As some ADRs are so rare a drug may need to be given to 10,000 or even 100,000 patients to pick up one incidence, or some drugs may need to be chronically administered for a long period, in order for an ADR to manifest. This is why reporting of ADRs is very important. All prescribers have a responsibility to report a potential ADR to the proper authorities. In the UK, the Committee for the Safety of Medicines (CSM) collects data and reports of ADRs. Reporting an ADR to the CSM can be done via the Yellow Card

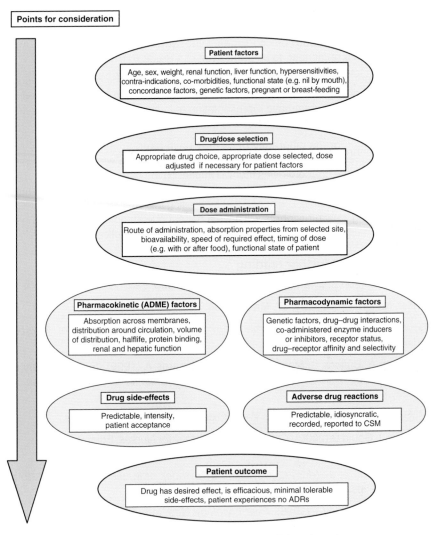

Points for consideration

Patient factors
Age, sex, weight, renal function, liver function, hypersensitivities, contra-indications, co-morbidities, functional state (e.g. nil by mouth), concordance factors, genetic factors, pregnant or breast-feeding

Drug/dose selection
Appropriate drug choice, appropriate dose selected, dose adjusted if necessary for patient factors

Dose administration
Route of administration, absorption properties from selected site, bioavailability, speed of required effect, timing of dose (e.g. with or after food), functional state of patient

Pharmacokinetic (ADME) factors
Absorption across membranes, distribution around circulation, volume of distribution, halflife, protein binding, renal and hepatic function

Pharmacodynamic factors
Genetic factors, drug–drug interactions, co-administered enzyme inducers or inhibitors, receptor status, drug–receptor affinity and selectivity

Drug side-effects
Predictable, intensity, patient acceptance

Adverse drug reactions
Predictable, idiosyncratic, recorded, reported to CSM

Patient outcome
Drug has desired effect, is efficacious, minimal tolerable side-effects, patient experiences no ADRs

Figure 7.9   Schematic representation for individualising drug therapy

system and yellow reporting cards can be found at the back of the BNF and joint Nurse Prescribers' Formulary (NPF)/BNF. The CSM collates information on ADRs from Yellow Card reporting and from other sources and then publish warnings and advice for prescribers to note about certain types of ADRs and how to minimise these. The CSM may also take the decision to revoke a licence and withdraw a drug from the market, if it is felt to be in the public's best interest.

INDIVIDUALISING DRUG THERAPY

In the previous four sections of this chapter, we have considered the basic principles and concepts with which prescribers should be familiar in order to prescribe safely and effectively. A lot of the issues covered will be considered almost sub-consciously by prescribers, e.g. in what form to administer a drug to a patient, other issues may need more considered thought e.g. does this patient's age require me, as a prescriber, to alter the dose of a drug?

What is important is that for every patient prescribed for, the prescriber should take an individual approach. No two patients will be alike and prescribers need to remember this. A diagrammatic representation of individualising drug therapy and the many issues that prescibers need to consider is shown in Figure 7.9.

Patients handle drugs differently once they have been administered and even when a drug reaches its site of action its effect may not be what was predicted. Patients may have co-morbidities that will impact on the expected drug effect; they may be taking other drugs that will interact; they may experience an ADR that may or may not be predictable. It is hoped that by reading this chapter and the suggested further reading, new prescribers will have a better understanding of some of these basic principles and consider them appropriately in their practice.

References and further reading

Bhalla *et al.* (2003). *Pharmaceutical Journal* **270**: 583–586.

British National Formulary, 47: March 2004.

Downie G *et al.* (1999). *Pharmacology and Drug Management for Nurses.* Edinburgh: Churchill Livingstone.

Galbraith A, Bullock S, Manias E, Hunt B, Richards A (1999). *Fundamentals of Pharmacology: A Text for Nurses and Health Professionals.* Harlow: Addison Wesley Longman.

McGavock H (2003). *How Drugs Work.* Oxford: Radcliffe Medical Press.

Trounce J, Gould D (2000). *Clinical Pharmacology for Nurses.* Edinburgh: Churchill Livingstone.

Weatherall DJ *et al.* (eds) (2003). *Oxford Textbook of Medicine.* Oxford: Oxford University Press.

Winstanley P, Walley T (1996). *Pharmacology.* New York: Churchill Livingstone.

Chapter 8

Monitoring skills

Part 1 – Asthma

Trisha Weller

INTRODUCTION

Asthma is common in the UK, with over 5 million asthma sufferers, and more than 3 million receiving current treatment (National Asthma Campaign (NAC), 2001). The prevalence of asthma has risen significantly over the last 25 years (British Thoracic Society (BTS), 2001) with the majority of asthma patients cared for within the primary care.

ASTHMA – THE DISEASE

Asthma is a reversible airways disease characterised by bronchoconstriction, inflammation, oedema and mucus production. It is reversible either spontaneously or with anti-asthma treatment.

The estimated prevalence rate of asthma in young children varies from 12.5% to 15.5%, while in adults current symptomatic asthma is reported by 7.8% adults (NAC, 2001). There is a wide spectrum of disease severity, and treatment requirements vary. Control of asthma is assessed against a standard of:

- minimal or no symptoms,
- minimal or no need for reliever medication,
- no exacerbations,
- no limitation of physical activity,
- normal lung function.

The British Guideline on the Management of Asthma (BTS/Scottish Intercollegiate Guidelines Network (SIGN), 2004) provides a framework for asthma treatment which is divided into treatment steps. These guidelines are further divided into age groups of:

- <5 years,
- 5–12 years,
- adults.

NURSE INVOLVEMENT IN ASTHMA MANAGEMENT

Many primary-care-based nurses have been involved with asthma management since the General Medical Services contract (Department of Health (DoH) and Social Security (DHSS), 1990) and the Health of the Nation White Paper (DoH, 1992), where payment was made to general practitioners for chronic disease management clinics and health promotion activities. In primary care, many of the responsibilities of chronic disease management, including asthma, have transferred to the practice nurse. Consequently, it is essential that these nurses have had appropriate asthma training. The British Guideline on the Management of Asthma (BTS/SIGN, 2004) which is an evidence-based guideline, states that '*In primary care, people with asthma should be reviewed regularly by a nurse or doctor with appropriate training in asthma management.*' The NAC, in their Asthma Charter 2003, supports the right of patients to have an access to a doctor or nurse who has had specific asthma training (www.asthma.org.uk).

The National Respiratory Training Centre (www.nrtc.org.uk), is the leading respiratory education provider for primary care nurses in the UK and more than 11,000 nurses have successfully completed their accredited diploma level asthma module. As a result, this asthma module is frequently a stated requirement for practice nurses and many have considerable knowledge and clinical skills in asthma management.

The British Guideline on the Management of Asthma (BTS/SIGN) has helped to standardise asthma care by defining a clinical management pathway based on published research evidence. New episodes of asthma are reported to be declining (Fleming *et al.*, 2000) and it has been suggested that nurses have contributed to this decline (Weller *et al.*, 2001).

GENERAL MEDICAL SERVICES CONTRACT

The new General Medical Services Contract (DoH, 2003) for primary care will reward general practices financially if they provide a quality health service. There are 10 clinical domains that will qualify for payment, including asthma and chronic obstructive pulmonary disease. One of the quality indicators within the asthma domain requires a review of asthma patients within the last 15 months. Similarly, within an organisational domain of medicines management, patients who are prescribed repeat medications should have a documented review of their medications. Accepted good asthma care is that patients with asthma should have their asthma medication requirements reviewed regularly, and stepped down to the minimum needed to control asthma symptoms (BTS, 2004).

ASTHMA TREATMENT PRIOR TO SUPPLEMENTARY PRESCRIBING

Prior to supplementary prescribing, many nurses involved in asthma management were already making treatment decisions. They assessed the asthma patient by:

- taking a detailed clinical history;
- performing diagnostic tests, such as a reversibility test;
- planning potential treatment with the patient, taking into account current asthma guidelines.

Discussion would take place with the general practitioner about suggested treatment. The doctors usually agreed and would sign the prescription the nurse had already prepared! In some situations, asthma-trained nurses may have had a more current asthma knowledge than their medical colleagues. Asthma management was based on the nurse's knowledge and clinical experience of asthma, and the support and trust of medical colleagues.

Nurses involved in asthma chronic disease management were frustrated by early prescribing restrictions. The introduction of independent prescribing allowed appropriately trained nurses to prescribe for both rhinitis and eczema (part of the atopic spectrum which includes asthma) as part of defined minor ailments (Medicines Control Agency (MCA), 2002). This meant that independent nurse prescribers could prescribe for their asthma patients if they also had eczema and rhinitis, but not for their asthma treatment.

SUPPLEMENTARY PRESCRIBING AND ASTHMA

Patients with asthma can now be assessed, reviewed and have their asthma medications prescribed by the supplementary prescriber (SP). The initial diagnosis needs to be confirmed by an independent prescriber (IP) who is a doctor. A clinical management plan (CMP) must be agreed by the IP and SP before supplementary prescribing begins, with the patient also agreeing and having an active role in this decision-making process. The British Guideline on the Management of Asthma provides evidence that an individual written asthma action plan (or self-management plan) detailing asthma treatment improves asthma outcomes (BTS/SIGN, 2004).

Although specific training in the clinical management of asthma is not a requirement of supplementary prescribing, there is evidence that an asthma-trained nurse can make a difference to clinical asthma outcomes (Dickinson *et al.*, 1997; BTS/SIGN, 2004). Therefore, it is likely that an asthma-trained supplementary nurse prescriber will provide a better asthma service than one who is not asthma trained.

PHARMACISTS AND ASTHMA MONITORING

Community pharmacists have an important role in monitoring asthma patients too, because they are often initially consulted for symptoms such as coughs and colds, and for 'over the counter' treatments. Colds can make asthma worse and a greater awareness of asthma monitoring and clinical management can enhance patient care. Pharmacists are eligible to become SPs but need to complete an accredited training education and training programme. A prescribing partnership must be established with a medical practitioner and shared records are essential. The need of pharmacists to acquire sound clinical asthma management skills is an area that needs addressing, in order to maintain optimum asthma care for patients.

How the role of supplementary prescribing pharmacist develops will not be known for sometime. However, potential developments could be their inclusion in the chronic disease management of patients with asthma or medication review clinics. These are likely to occur in both primary and secondary care. Other developments are likely to follow with the development of the new pharmacists contract. These may include the 'sub-contracting' of services from community pharmacists to Primary Care Trusts (PCTs) to develop clinics, potentially allowing more choice to the patient.

ASTHMA MEDICATIONS

There are three main groups of asthma medications. They are:

- bronchodilators,
- glucocorticosteroids,
- leukotriene receptor antagonists (LTRAs).

BRONCHODILATORS

These are divided into:

1. Short-acting bronchodilators (β 2 agonists), e.g. salbutamol, terbutaline.
2. Anti-cholinergic medications, e.g. ipratropium bromide.
3. Long-acting bronchodilators, e.g. salmeterol and formoterol.
4. Methylxanthines, e.g. theophyllines and aminophylline.

Short-acting bronchodilators: these are used for symptomatic relief on an as required basis for wheeze, cough, breathlessness, and chest tightness. They are used in high doses in worsening and acute asthma. Common side-effects are tachycardia and tremor and are usually dose related.

Anti-cholinergic medication: ipratropium bromide, is used for the treatment of acute severe asthma where there has been an initial poor response to short-acting bronchodilators. It is nebulised with short-acting bronchodilators (BTS/SIGN, 2004). Side-effects include a dry mouth.

Long-acting bronchodilators: these are used as first-line-additional therapy to short-acting bronchodilators and low dose corticosteroids. They should not be used to treat an acute asthma attack. Side-effects are similar to short-acting bronchodilators.

Methylxanthines: these are used as additional therapy when there is no response to the long-acting bronchodilator therapy. There is wide variability in the half-life of the drug. It is increased in heart failure, cirrhosis, viral infections, and the elderly, and by drugs such as cimetidine, ciprofloxacin, erythromycin, and oral contraceptives. It is decreased in smokers and chronic alcoholism and by drugs such as phenytoin, carbamazepine, rifampicin and barbiturates. There is a narrow therapeutic safety window for methylxanthines and regular blood monitoring should be instigated because of the potential for side-effects, such as tachycardia, gastrointestinal disturbance, headache, insomnia, and convulsions.

GLUCOCORTICOSTEROIDS

There are four inhaled glucocorticosteroids available in the UK:

- Beclometasone
- Budesonide
- Fluticasone
- Mometasone.

Inhaled steroids are the first-line preventer therapy for asthma (BTS/SIGN, 2004). The lowest dose possible should be used to control asthma symptoms. Local side-effects of dysphonia and candidiasis occur rarely but are usually dose related. Systemic side-effects are very rare in lower-dose ranges (up to 800 micrograms beclomethasone dipropionate (BDP) or equivalent). Inhaled steroids need to be taken regularly to obtain maximum benefit.

It is important to remember that fluticasone is used at half the dose of beclometasone or budesonide. Several reports indicate the likelihood of more serious side-effects of adrenal insufficiency at doses above 500 micrograms fluticasone per day (Todd et al., 1996; 2002). Current BTS/SIGN (BTS/SIGN, 2004) guidelines suggest an upper limit of 800 micrograms beclometasone or equivalent.

Hawkins et al. (2003) report that inhaled steroids can be reduced effectively in patients with moderate to severe asthma without compromising asthma control. This study supports current guideline recommendations that lower doses of inhaled steroids should be used. Health professionals monitoring asthma patients need to ensure that asthma review includes reducing asthma treatment to the minimum needed to control symptoms.

Steroid cards are not issued routinely to asthma patients on inhaled corticosteroids but those taking regular oral steroids must be issued with one. Supplies of these cards are available from the DoH.

LEUKOTRIENE RECEPTOR ANTAGONISTS

LTRAs are oral therapies that are generally used in addition to inhaled steroids and following a trial of long-acting bronchodilators. In children from ages 6 months–5 years, they can be used as first-line preventer therapy. There are two products available in the UK – montelukast and zafirlukast. Montelukast is used more widely and is taken once daily at night. Side-effects include gastrointestinal disturbances and dry mouth.

ASTHMA MEDICATIONS AND PREGNANCY

Asthma patients who are pregnant should be treated the same way as those who are not pregnant. Asthma medications should be continued in pregnancy including the use of oral steroids if they are required. LTRAs are not indicated in pregnancy unless prior treatment has demonstrated them to be clinically effective (BTS/SIGN, 2004).

ASTHMA MEDICATIONS IN YOUNG CHILDREN

Several asthma medications are unlicensed for the younger paediatric asthma patient because of the ages defined within the product licence. The Royal College of Paediatricians and Child Health (RCPCH) have published a policy statement on the use of unlicensed medicines, or licensed medicines for unlicensed applications in paediatric practice (RCPCH, 2003). The use of these medicines can be justified where it is the most appropriate medication, but parents of these children must be informed as to why this choice was made.

There are several drug strengths available for many of the different asthma medications, as well as a range of drug-delivery systems. The higher drug strengths are not indicated for children over 12 years, but this raises the question as to 'what age defines a child?'. Licensing applications need to be more specific to avoid potential confusion for prescribers. Table 8.1 illustrates the variable licensing age ranges of inhaled steroids and long-acting bronchodilators.

Table 8.1   Licensing age ranges for inhaled steroids and long-acting bronchodilators

Drug	Age range
Beclometasone	From 6 months
Budesonide	Birth onwards
Fluticasone	4 years and over
250 micrograms Accuhaler device	Not indicated for children
500 micrograms Accuhaler device	Not indicated for children
250 micrograms Diskhaler device	Not indicated for children
500 micrograms Diskhaler device	Not indicated for children
125 micrograms Evohaler device	Not indicated for children
250 micrograms Evohaler device	Not indicated for children
Mometasone	12 years and over
Salmeterol	4 years and over
Formoterol	From 6 years via Turbohaler device; 5 years via other dry powder device

Source: British National Formulary (BNF), September 2003.

Table 8.2 illustrates the variable licensing ages for combination therapy of inhaled steroid and long-acting bronchodilators. This variability can lead to confusion for prescribers where the separate components have different licensing age ranges.

There is considerable variability in licensing age ranges for asthma medications. When new products first appear on the market, licensing indications are usually restricted to 12 years and over. This age range relates to the research studies carried out to obtain a product license. It does not mean that the products are unsafe below the stated age range; merely there are no supporting studies when the product was first licensed.

Nurses monitoring asthma patients need to be aware not only of the medication required, according to current guidelines, but also product license indications.

MONITORING ADVERSE EFFECTS

Nurses can now report drug side-effects using the established Yellow Card system (Committee on Safety of Medicine (CSM)/MCA, 2002). This drug reporting system provides an early warning system to the Medicines and Healthcare products Regulatory Agency (MHRA) (previously known as the MCA and the CSM). The Yellow Card reporting system began in 1964 after the drug thalidomide was withdrawn, but reporting was limited to doctors, dentists, coroners and pharmacists, as well as the pharmaceutical industry. Inclusion of nurses within the current reporting system acknowledges the important monitoring role that nurses have in drug usage, especially within chronic disease management. Electronic submission is also possible, which facilitates easier and quicker submission of reports.

Newly licensed medications are monitored carefully by the MHRA and the CSM when they are first introduced or if there is a change in drug-route or -delivery system.

Table 8.2   Variable drug doses and relevant licensing age for combination asthma therapies

Seretide (Fluticasone + salmeterol)	Age range
100 micrograms Accuhaler device	Over 4 years
250 micrograms Accuhaler device	Over 12 years
500 micrograms Accuhaler device	Over 12 years
50 micrograms Evohaler (metered dose inhaler)	Over 12 years*
125 micrograms Evohaler	Over 12 years
250 micrograms Evohaler	Over 12 years
Symbicort (Budesonide + formoterol)	Age range
100/6	Over 6 years
200/6	Over 12 years

Source: British National Formulary (BNF), September 2003.
*Now from age 4 years.

These medications are indicated by a black triangle symbol in the BNF and the Monthly Index of Medical Specialities (MIMS). No upper time limit is set for this black triangle identification but these medications are usually reviewed after a minimum of 2 years.

ASTHMA MONITORING

At each asthma review it is important to:

- Review any medication changes including dose alterations.
- Always ask the patient or carer what they are taking. This can be different to what has been prescribed.
- Be alert to possible medication side-effects.
- Assess inhaler technique and modify technique when appropriate.
- Change inhaler device if technique cannot be corrected.
- Consider the addition of a spacer device if high doses of inhaled steroid are used.
- Treatment should follow national asthma guideline recommendations.
- Provide a written action plan tailored to the individual (BTS/SIGN, 2004) and agreed with the independent medical prescriber and asthma patient.
- Issue a peak flow meter and determine appropriate peak flow values with the patient as part of the asthma action plan, for those with:
  - brittle or life-threatening asthma,
  - previous admissions to hospital,
  - unscheduled care for asthma emergencies,
  - frequent courses of oral steroids,
  - treatment at step 3 Asthma Guidelines (BTS/SIGN, 2004) and above.
- Provide a follow up review date.

SUMMARY

Supplementary prescribing will enhance the care that asthma patients receive. Monitoring of respiratory symptoms and drug therapy is essential but should be carried out by a health professional who has established expertise in asthma management and national asthma guidelines should be followed. A multidisciplinary approach to care is essential.

FURTHER INFORMATION

Asthma Training. Further information is available from the National Respiratory Training Centre. www.nrtc.org.uk. Enquiries: Tel: 01926 493313.

Asthma UK (Previously National Asthma Campaign.) www.asthma.org.uk

British Guideline on the Management of Asthma. www.brit-thoracic.org.uk

STEROID CARDS ARE AVAILABLE FROM

DoH, PO Box 777, London SE1 6XH

Scotland: South Gyle Crescent, Edinburgh EH12 9EB

References (asthma)

BTS (2001). *The Burden of Lung Disease. A Statistics Report from the British Thoracic Society.*

BTS/SIGN (2004). *British Guideline on the Management of Asthma.* Revised ed. Edinburgh: SIGN. (SIGN Publication no 63). [cited 20 April 2004]. Available from url: http://www.sign.ac.uk/guidelines/fulltext/63/index.html

CSM/MCA (2002). *Extension of the Yellow Card Scheme to Nurse Reporters.*

DoH (1992). *The Health of the Nation: A Strategy for Health in England,* London: HMSO.

DoH (2003). *Investing in General Practice: The New General Medical Services Contract.* London: DoH.

DHSS (1990). *General Practice in the National Health Service. A New Contract.* London: HMSO.

Dickinson J, Hutton S, Atkin A *et al.* (1997). Reducing asthma morbidity in the community: the effect of a targeted nurse-run asthma clinic in an English general practice. *Respiratory Medicine* **91**: 634–640.

Fleming DM, Sunderland R, Cross KW, Ross AM (2000). Declining incidence of episodes of asthma: a study of trends in new episodes presenting to general practitioners in the period 1989–1998. *Thorax* **55(8)**: 657–661.

Hawkins G, McMahon AD, Twaddle S, Wood SF, Ford I, Thompson NC (2003). Stepping down inhaled corticosteroids in asthma: a randomised controlled trial. *British Medical Journal* **326**: 1115–1118.

MCA (2002). *Proposals for Supplementary Prescribing by Nurses and Pharmacist and Proposed Amendments to the Prescription Only Medicines (Human use) Order 1997* MLX 284.

National Asthma Campaign (NAC) (2001). Out in the open. *Asthma Journal* **6(3)** (**suppl**): 1–14.

Royal College of Paediatricians and Child Health (2003). The use of unlicensed medicines or licensed medicines for unlicensed applications in paediatric practice. In: *Medicines for Children* 2nd edn. London: RCPCH Publications Limited, pp. xvi–xviii.

Todd G, Dunlop K, McNaboe J, Ryan MF, Carson D, Shields MD (1996). Growth and adrenal suppression in asthmatic children treated with high-dose fluticasone propionate. *Lancet* **348**: 27–29.

Todd GRG, Acerini CL, Buck JJ, Murphy NP, Ross-Russell R, Warner JT, McCance DR (2002). Acute adrenal crisis in asthmatics treated with high-dose fluticasone propionate. *European Respiratory Journal* **19**: 1207–1209.

Weller T, Booker R, Walker S (2001). Declining incidence of episodes of asthma: letter. *Thorax* **56(3)**: 246.

Part 2 – Coronary heart disease

Paul Warburton

INTRODUCTION

Coronary heart disease (CHD) is the leading cause of mortality in the developed world. In the UK diseases of the heart and circulatory system are the main cause of death, accounting for 240,000 deaths in 2001 (British Heart Foundation (BHF), 2003). CHD is the most common cause of death in the UK, killing over 120,000 people in 2001, up to 70,000 of these before the age of 75 (BHF). Despite recent reductions, the death rate from CHD in the UK remains amongst the highest in the world.

CHD is a common condition that has a significant impact on the individual; it is frequently fatal and often debilitating, leading to a reduction in the quality of life. The economic cost to society is enormous; CHD is estimated to cost the UK economy a total of £7055 million annually (Liu *et al.*, 1999), yet it is largely preventable. The underlying pathology of CHD is usually atherosclerosis and this develops over many years, often without any signs or symptoms. In men, the first indication of CHD is often myocardial infarction (40%) or death (13%) (Deedwania, 2001).

There are a number of well-recognised and understood risk factors for CHD, and the modification of these risk factors has been conclusively shown to reduce mortality and morbidity in both individuals with or without a previous history of CHD. Risk factors can be categorised as fixed or modifiable (Table 8.3). The fixed risk factors of age, male sex or a family history of CHD cannot be corrected.

When discussing the risk of developing a condition such as CHD, it is important to distinguish between relative risk (the proportional increase in risk) and the absolute risk (the actual chance of an event). The risk of developing CHD multiplies when there is more than one risk factor present. Therefore, people with a combination of risk factors have a greater risk of developing CHD. For example, a man of 40 who smokes 30 cigarettes per day and has an elevated cholesterol level of 8 mmol/l, is far more likely to die in the next 10 years from CHD than a non-smoking woman of the same age, with a low cholesterol level. However, the likelihood of this happening is still low. He, therefore, has a high relative risk of developing CHD but low absolute risk.

Table 8.3   Risk factors for CHD

Fixed	Modifiable
Age	Smoking
Male sex	Hypertension
Family history	Raised cholesterol
	Diabetes
	Obesity
	Sedentary lifestyle

FIXED RISK FACTORS

The risk of an individual developing CHD rises with age and males are affected in larger numbers than females. Family history is an important fixed risk factor; the Framingham study (Schildkraut *et al.*, 1989) has shown that a history of death due to CHD in parents of an individual, was associated with a 30% increased risk of developing CHD. This may be due to genetic factors or the effects of a shared environment, (such as a similar diet) and habits (such as smoking). As CHD often runs in families, the first-degree relatives of patients with premature CHD (men <55 years and women <65 years) and those with family members who have hyperlipidaemia, should be risk assessed for developing CHD and treated as appropriate.

MODIFIABLE RISK FACTORS

Smoking

Smoking is probably the most avoidable cause of CHD. There is a strong, consistent and dose-related relationship between cigarette smoking and CHD. It promotes the build-up of coronary plaques and can lead to premature plaque rupture and subsequent myocardial infarction. It is estimated that about 20% of deaths in men and 17% in women are due to smoking. Yet, despite the recognised relationship between smoking and CHD, in 2000, 29% of men and 25% of women smoked in the UK (BHF, 2003).

Hypertension

In western societies, the average systolic and diastolic blood pressure rises with age. In England 40% of men and 39% of women have hypertension, or are being treated for hypertension (BHF, 2003). Hypertension is defined as a systolic blood pressure of 140 mmHg or over or a diastolic blood pressure of 90 mmHg or over. The risk of developing CHD and other vascular disorders is related directly to both systolic and diastolic blood pressure levels (National Heart Forum, 2002). The risk of developing vascular disease associated with hypertension rises continuously across the pressure ranges. Therefore, a reduction in blood pressure leads to a decreased risk of not only CHD but also other circulatory conditions such as stroke and renal dysfunction.

In more than 95% of cases of hypertension, no underlying cause is found. This is known as essential hypertension. In 70% of those with essential hypertension, another family member is affected.

Hypertension is diagnosed following the measurement of blood pressure on three separate occasions. A patient with an isolated episode of recorded hypertension (isolated systolic hypertension $\geqslant$160 mmHg) is associated with an increased risk of stroke and coronary events, and should be kept under review. In the majority of cases, the discovery of hypertension will mean a lifetime of monitoring and treatment with antihypertensive medications. However, general lifestyle measurements can prove to be successful in the reduction of blood pressure. Reduction in alcohol consumption, reducing salt intake and correcting obesity are effective in reducing blood pressure levels. Regular exercise improves physical conditioning and can also lead to a lower blood pressure.

Diet and obesity

Consumption of a 'healthy' diet is associated with a reduced risk of developing cardiovascular and other diseases. Such a diet has benefits of maintaining appropriate weight, reducing plasma lipids and lowering blood pressure. This can help to reduce the risk of developing CHD. Recommendations include a reduction in fat intake, particularly saturated fats, reduction in salt intake and an increase in the intake of carbohydrates, and fruit and vegetables (Department of Health (DoH), 1994). It is with this in mind that the DoH have introduced the current 'five a day' recommendations of five portions of fruit and vegetables each day. The number of people who are overweight or obese in the UK is increasing and has roughly doubled since the mid-1980s; this is probably due to increasing calorific intake and increased sedentary lifestyles within the population. Obesity is associated with other cardiovascular risk factors, such as hypertension and diabetes. Worryingly, 79% of men and 71% of women aged 55–64 in the UK are overweight or obese (Joint Health Surveys Units (JHSU), 1999). The incidence of type 2 diabetes due to insulin resistance is associated with obesity, is common in this age group and is a strong risk factor for the development of CHD.

Diabetes

Diabetes is a common disorder that affects approximately 1.4 million people in the UK, with around 90% of these having type 2 diabetes (BHF, 2001). Patients with diabetes have a 2 to 3-fold increased risk of having a CHD event – the relative risk is higher in women. This is similar to the risk of non-diabetics with established CHD (Haffner et al., 1998). The primary prevention of CHD and assessment and treatment of risk in diabetics is, therefore, essential and this patient group benefits from being treated as if they have existing CHD. The benefits of rigorous blood pressure control in diabetics has been demonstrated in the United Kingdom Prospective Diabetes Study (UKPDS) Study Group (1998).

Hypercholesterolaemia

There is evidence that the risk of developing CHD is directly related to blood cholesterol levels. Target levels for blood cholesterol are 5 mmol/l for total cholesterol and

3 mmol/l for low density lipoprotein cholesterol (LDL-C). Lowering the concentration of both total cholesterol and LDL-C is effective in the primary and secondary prevention of CHD.

RISK CALCULATORS

There are a large number of well-recognised cardiovascular risk calculator tools available to calculate the absolute risk of developing CHD. These include the Joint British Societies Coronary Risk Prediction Chart (Wood *et al.*, 1998) which can be found in the back of the BNF (2003) and the European Society of Cardiology's Score system (2003). These are primary prevention aids and are tools for estimating the risk of developing CHD for individuals who have not already developed CHD.

Risk calculators are a useful aid to clinical decision-making when considering pharmacological intervention, such as lipid-lowering or antihypertensive therapy. They are also valuable in illustrating to patients the benefits of risk factor modification, such as stopping smoking or a reduction in cholesterol levels.

Risk calculators provide a 10-year risk of developing CHD and this is expressed as a percentage figure. Higher risk individuals are defined as those whose 10-year risk of developing CHD exceeds 15% and the highest risk classified is greater than 30%. They should be used as a decision-making tool and should not replace clinical judgement.

MEDICATIONS USED IN PRIMARY PREVENTION OF CORONARY HEART DISEASE

When prescribing medications to reduce the risk of CHD the principles of good prescribing apply. It is important to discuss with patients the treatment options available to address their individual risk factors. The purpose, effects and possible side-effects of the medication(s) should be explained along with how and when it should be taken. The alternatives to the prescribed treatment should also be discussed.

Antihypertensives

The purpose of treating hypertension is to lower blood pressure effectively, reduce the risk of complications and improve survival. Antihypertensives should reduce blood pressure and be well tolerated. There is a wide range of evidence-based medications available to treat hypertension; often, combination therapy of more than one medication is required to attain adequate blood pressure control. These are usually added in a stepwise manner until control is achieved. There are five classes of first-line drugs currently used to treat hypertension.

Thiazides

A low-dose thiazide is the first-line treatment for hypertension unless a contra-indication exists or there is a specific indication for another class of drug. May take up to 4 weeks for the maximum effect to be observed.

Beta-blockers

Are effective antihypertensive agents, especially when used in combination with a thiazide. They are available in large numbers and are widely used for a number of cardiovascular conditions. However, they may cause unwanted side-effects and are contraindicated in asthmatics.

ACE-Inhibitors

These are very effective antihypertensives. They inhibit the conversion of angiotensin 1 to angiotensin 2 and have a good side-effect profile. The most common side-effect is a dry persistent cough. Angiotensin-converting enzyme-inhibitors (ACE-I) should be used with care in patients with impaired renal function. Urea and creatinine levels should be monitored in all patients before commencing an ACE-I and 7–10 days after starting or increasing the dose.

Calcium channel blockers

There are different actions and effects of calcium channel blockers, they all interfere with the inward displacement of calcium ions through the cell membranes. They are usually well tolerated some side-effects such as flushing, headache and ankle swelling can occur.

Angiotensin II receptor antagonists

These have an action similar to that of the ACE-Inhibitors but do not cause the persistent dry cough that is associated with the ACE-I. Currently there is little evidence to suggest benefit over using an ACE-I. As with ACE-I these should be used with care in patients with impaired renal function and urea and creatinine levels should be monitored in all patients before commencing and 7–10 days after starting an Angiotensin II receptor antagonists (AIIAs).

Antiplatelet medications

Antiplatelet medications reduce platelet aggregation in the arterial circulation and may inhibit thrombus formation. There is evidence that the use of aspirin in people who do not have established vascular disease reduces the risk of myocardial infarction but does not reduce the risk of stroke (Hart *et al.*, 2000). In asymptomatic high-risk individuals, a low dose of aspirin is beneficial in the primary prevention of CHD when the 10-year risk is greater than 15%.

Cholesterol lowering medications

There are a number of medications available to reduce cholesterol levels. These include statins, fibrates and anion-exchange resins. Statins are the first choice and are now the mainstay of cholesterol-lowering treatment, in both the primary and secondary prevention of CHD. There are a number of effective statins available with varying degrees of potency. They competitively inhibit an enzyme involved in the synthesis of cholesterol called 3-hydroxy-3-methylglutaryl coenzyme A (HMG CoA) reductase. There is conclusive evidence of their ability to reduce both primary and secondary cardiovascular events.

Smoking

Smoking cessation interventions can reduce ill health and prolong life and are cost effective. Nicotine replacement therapy (NRT) and bupropion are effective aids to smoking cessation in individuals who are motivated to stop, and who smoke more than 10 cigarettes each day. The success of such therapies is increased when supported by a clinic (Rice, 2003). The British National Formulary (BNF) includes a useful overview on the subject of smoking cessation.

Nicotine replacement products are P-Category medications and as such are able to be purchased over the counter with advice from a Pharmacist. They can also be prescribed by District Nurse/Health Visitor prescribers and Extended Formulary Nurse Prescribers. Bupropion could be included in a Clinical Management Plan (CMP) and therefore could be prescribed by a SP.

THE NATIONAL SERVICE FRAMEWORK AND PRIMARY PREVENTION

The National Service Framework (NSF) for CHD (DoH, 2000) suggests that individuals without diagnosed CHD who have a risk of greater than 30% of developing CHD over 10 years, should be identified and structured care provided, to reduce their risk of CHD. In such individuals, the following steps should be taken:

- Smokers should be advised to give up and be supported with appropriate intervention, such as NRT.
- A healthy lifestyle should be promoted. Assessment of individual risk factors should be made and information given, as appropriate, regarding modifiable risk factors for such as diet, physical activity, weight, alcohol consumption and where applicable diabetes control. Information should be personalised to individual needs.
- Where blood pressure exceeds 140/80, advice and treatment to maintain blood pressure below this level should be given (see below).
- A statin should be added to lower serum cholesterol to <5 mmol/l and LDL-C to <3 mmol/l.

For patients with diabetes, blood glucose levels should be well-controlled and the treatment goals for blood pressure and cholesterol control should be lower, e.g. blood pressure $<140/80$ mmHg, total cholesterol <4.5 mmol/l and LDL-C <2.5 mmol/l (Backer, 2003).

INDIVIDUAL RISK ASSESSMENT

The assessment of the risk of an individual developing CHD should be performed and updated, at least every 5 years. This will allow the identification of those at greatest risk. This will include those patients with a family history of premature CHD or hyperlipidaemia and patients with hypertension or diabetes. This assessment can be done opportunistically in primary care when a patient attends an appointment with a doctor, nurse or pharmacist, or at a routine review, such as a repeat prescription review or new-patient screening. The following information should be gathered and recorded on a patient's health record:

- Blood pressure
- Height and weight/body mass index calculated
- Cholesterol levels
- Smoking habits
- Alcohol intake
- Diet
- History of significant risk factors, such as hypertension or diabetes
- Family history of premature CHD, diabetes, hypertension or cerebrovascular accident (CVA).

The identification of an individual as being at increased risk of developing CHD leads to many challenges for the individual and the nurse. Patterns of behaviour, such as smoking, a sedentary lifestyle and diet, are usually life-long and often require professional assistance in making change. Referral to other services, such as a dietician, may prove useful. Once lifestyle modification has taken place, and despite being asymptomatic, many patients will still need to take medications. Concordance with medications is therefore often a problem, particularly when polypharmacy is needed or if side-effects occur. The management of patients at high risk of developing CHD requires a collaborative approach to change and the benefits of these changes should be explained and reiterated to each patient.

References

British Heart Foundation (2003). *Coronary Heart Disease Statistics: British Heart Foundation Statistics Database.* London: British Heart Foundation.

British Heart Foundation (2001). *Coronary Heart Disease Statistics: Diabetes Supplement.* London: British Heart Foundation.

British Medical Association and the Royal Pharmaceutical Society of Great Britain. (2003). London: British National Formulary.

Guideline for the management of hypertension: report of the third working party of the British hypertension society (1999). *Journal Human Hypertension* **13**: 569–592.

Deedwania P (2001). Global risk assessment in the presymptomatic patient. *American Journal of Cardiology* **88(suppl)**: 17J–22J.

Department of Health (1994). *Nutritional Aspects of Cardiovascular Disease. Report of the Cardiovascular Review Group of the Committee on Medical Aspects of Food Policy.* London: HMSO.

European guidelines on cardiovascular disease prevention in clinical practice (2003). *European Heart Journal* **24**: 1601–1610.

Haffner SM, Lehto S, Ronnemaa T, Pyorala K, Laakso M (1998). Mortality from Coronary Heart Disease in subjects with type II diabetes and in non-diabetic subjects with and without prior myocardial infarction. *New England Journal Medicine* **339**: 229–234.

Hart RG, Halperin JL, McBride R, Benavente O, Man-Son-Hing M, Kronmal RA (2000). Aspirin for the primary prevention of stroke and other major vascular events. Meta-analysis and hypotheses. *Archives of Neurology* **57**: 326–332.

Joint Health Surveys Unit (1999). *Health Survey for England 1998*. London: The Stationery Office.

Liu JLY, Maniadakis N, Gray A, Rayner M (2002). The economic burden of coronary heart disease in the UK. *Heart* **88**: 597–603.

National Heart Forum (2003). *Coronary Heart Disease: Estimating the Impact of Change in Risk Factors*. London: The Stationery Office.

Rice VH, Stead LF (2003). Nursing interventions for smoking cessation (Cochrane Methodology Review). In: *The Cochrane Library* Issue 4. Chichester, UK: John Wiley & Sons, Ltd.

Schildkraut JM, Myers RH, Cupples LA, Kiely DK, Kannel WB (1989). Aspirin for the primary prevention of stroke and other major vascular events. Meta-analysis and hypotheses. *Archives of Neurology* **57**: 326–332.

United Kingdom Prospective Diabetes Study Group (1998). Intensive blood glucose control with sulphonylurea or insulin compared with conventional treatment and risk of complications in type 2 diabetes (UKPDS 34). *Lancet* **352**: 854–865.

Wood D, Durrington P, Poulter N, McInnes G, Rees A, Wray A (1998). Joint British recommendations on prevention of coronary heart disease in clinical practice. *Heart* **80(suppl 2)**: S1–S29.

Part 3 – Diabetes

Lesley Metcalfe

One of the principle aims of the extended independent and supplementary nurse prescribing programme is the potential to improve patient care by enabling faster access to medicine for people who have chronic medical conditions such as diabetes mellitus (Department of Health (DoH), 2002a). The profile of diabetes service delivery has increased following the publication of the National Service Framework (NSF) (DoH 2002b). The delivery strategy includes a recommendation to take advantage of nurse prescribing.

Diabetes is a chronic, lifelong condition that affects large numbers of people; there are an estimated 1.4 million known sufferers in the UK. Diabetes mellitus is a metabolic disorder characterised by chronic hyperglycaemia caused by defects in insulin secretion and action. Prolonged hyperglycaemia due to impaired insulin effects is associated with the development of microvascular and macrovascular complications, causing morbidity and premature mortality. Common complications of diabetes include retinopathy, neuropathy, nephropathy, angina, myocardial infarction, stroke and erectile dysfunction. People with diabetes can also suffer considerable anxiety relating to their condition, its management and uncertainties about long-term complications (National Institute of Clinical Excellence (NICE), 2003a).

TYPES OF DIABETES

Type 1

- Total insulin deficiency that tends to affect people below the age of 40 years

- Accounts for approximately 15–20% of diabetes

- Characterised by acute onset of symptoms which can only be treated with insulin therapy

- Life expectancy reduced by 20 years

(DoH, 2001a)

Type 2

- Impaired insulin secretion with insensitivity to target tissues to insulin; also known as insulin resistance

- Tends to manifest in later adult life

- Often diagnosed incidentally or because of the presence of diabetes related complications and accounts for 80–85% of diabetes

- The fourth leading cause of death in most developed countries

- Life expectancy reduced by 10 years

(DoH, 2001b)

Maturity onset of diabetes of the young

- Rare

- Usually diagnosed below the age of 25 years

- Inherited as an autosomal dominant gene

- Low susceptibility to complications

Gestational diabetes

- Pregnancy increases hormonal antagonists and insulin therapy may be required

- There is an increased risk of diabetes in later life (Diabetes UK, 2002)

Diabetes is progressive and sufferers will inevitably require a selection of medication to control symptoms initially and thereafter attain treatment goals in order to prevent the complications associated with this chronic condition.

The principal goal of treatment is to prevent acute complications of diabetes that can affect daily life, such as hypoglycaemia or hyperglycaemia and in the long-term, the prevention of complications. Evidence from landmark studies such as the Diabetes Control and Complications Trial (DCCT) and United Kingdom Prospective Diabetes Study (UKPDS) proves that early intensive management of diabetes and other risk factors such as blood pressure, lipid levels, weight management and lifestyle can achieve treatment goals.

The treatment goals now aimed at in practice have been derived from the strong evidence base that exists (UKPDS, 1998; European Guidelines, 2003).

Targets	
Glycosylated haemoglobin (HbA1c)	<7%
Fasting plasma glucose	<6.0 mmol/l
Blood pressure	<140/80
Total cholesterol	<4.5 mmol/l
LDL Cholesterol	<2.5 mmol/l

Treatment goals and targets can only be achieved by patient participation and compliance with treatment regimes. Regular monitoring of progress, combined with appropriate and timely intervention by healthcare professionals in primary care, or by specialist diabetes teams in secondary care, is essential to stay a step ahead of the progressive condition that is diabetes. The role of the diabetes specialist nurse (DSN) is viewed as pivotal in helping people with diabetes achieve treatment goals by providing continuity and advice tailored to individual needs (Thynne *et al.*, 2003).

Supplementary prescribing provides an opportunity to further enhance the role of the DSN and involve pharmacist colleagues working in primary and secondary care to improve service delivery. In particular, supplementary prescribing, which requires a patient-specific clinical management plan (CMP) to be agreed between the patient concerned and the independent prescriber (IP), will enable the DSN or specialist pharmacist to modify diabetes therapies in a timely fashion. This will also complement the NSF requirement that all patients have a care plan. This may improve concordance, defined as an '*agreement reached after negotiation between patient and healthcare professional ... in treatment decisions*' (DoH, 2001c). The care plan will enable the patient to review the agreement and make appropriate changes to improve their diabetes control.

Monitoring of diabetes therapy regimes must begin at diagnosis, to enable the person with diabetes to be fully informed and have an understanding of what to expect.

Education is considered to be a fundamental element of the diabetes care provided by diabetes care teams in both primary and secondary care settings (NICE, 2003b). The aim of education for people with diabetes, regardless of treatment regimes, is to empower them with the knowledge and skills to manage the condition. Involvement in the early stages will encourage commitment and compliance. Diabetes education should be tailored to suit individual needs, but should include information about what diabetes is, monitoring techniques, treatment regimes, life style issues and the importance of regular review.

TREATMENT REGIMES

Diet

Diet is the cornerstone of diabetes management, regardless of the type of diabetes. A healthy, balanced diet, low in glucose and saturated fats and high in fibre, underpins treatment regimes. Individually tailored advice should be given by a dietician, to all newly diagnosed people, with the opportunity for review as needs dictate. All members of the diabetes care team have a role to play by reinforcing dietary advice given. A new concept is a structured educational programme, the dose adjustment for normal eating (DAFNE), and is aimed at people with type 1 diabetes, which allows for enhanced dietary freedom by teaching insulin adjustment to match carbohydrate intake on a meal-by-meal basis.

INSULIN THERAPY

There are many types of insulin therapy, regimes and delivery devices available today. The choice of insulin preparation will depend on:

- Type of diabetes
- Lifestyle
- Individual choice
- Ability to administer insulin independently.

Types of insulin

Rapid-acting insulin analogues: are the new generation of shorter-acting insulins and include Insulin Aspart (NovoRapid) and Insulin Lispro (Humalog). They are clear preparations that start to act within 5–15 minutes of injection, and are usually administered at meal times three times per day, in combination with a bedtime injection of intermediate or long-acting insulin.

Available in vial, cartridge and disposable pen device, they can also be used as a continuous subcutaneous infusion via an insulin pump.

Short-acting insulins: Include Human Actrapid, Humulin S and Insuman Rapid, they are clear preparations which should be administered 20–30 minutes before eating. They can be used as a multiple injection regime as above or as a twice-daily regime in combination with an intermediate or long-acting insulin. These are available in vial, cartridges and disposable pen devices.

Intermediate-acting insulins: are Isophane insulins and include Human Insulatard, Humulin I and Insuman Basal. They are cloudy preparations that provide longer action of up to 16 hours. They are used as part of a multiple injection regime, given once at bedtime or in combination with a short-acting insulin given twice daily with breakfast and evening meal. They are available in vial, cartridge and as a disposable pen device.

Long-acting insulin analogue: Only recently available in the UK, Insulin Glargine (Lantus) is a clear preparation, which is designed to last for 24 hours without peaking. This flat profile is thought to reduce the risk of potential hypoglycaemia. This once daily injection can be used in combination with rapid acting and short-acting insulins as a multiple injection regime. Or it can be used as a once daily regime for type 2 diabetes, with or without oral hypoglycaemic agents (OHA). It is available in vial, cartridge and as a disposable pen device.

Long-acting insulins: include Monotard, Ultratard, Lente and Humulin ZN, they are cloudy preparations which work for 24 hours or more. They have the potential for causing hypoglycaemia due to their long action. They are available in vials for use with syringe, but are not usually the insulin of choice any more.

Biphasic insulins: are mixtures of rapid or short-acting insulin with intermediate insulin in various combinations and include Human Mixtard 10, 20, 30, 40, Humulin M2, M3, M5, Insuman Comb 15, 25, 50, NovoMix 30, and Humalog Mix 25 (the number indicates the amount of rapid- or short-acting insulin combination). They are injected twice daily at breakfast and evening meal times. They are cloudy preparations and are available in vial, cartridge and as disposable pen devices.

Animal insulins: are still available and include Hypurin Neutral, Hypurin Isophane and Hypurin 30/70 mix. Available in vial and cartridges, they are not usually prescribed for new patients today.

CONSIDERATIONS

Wherever possible, the person who requires insulin therapy to manage their Diabetes, should be given a choice as to the regime and delivery device to suit individual needs and lifestyle. Patient involvement from the beginning will encourage commitment and compliance and assist self-management (DoH, 2001a). Diabetes UK (2002) encourages healthcare professionals working in diabetes teams to personalise education to ensure success and lasting impact.

Injection technique

Injection technique, timing and the importance of injection site rotation are subjects generally discussed at insulin initiation. The choice of needle length and the method for disposal of sharps is included. Devices for the removal of sharps can be prescribed and include the NovoFine Remover and the BD Safeclip device.

ORAL HYPOGLYCAEMIC AGENTS

Initial management of type 2 diabetes generally begins with lifestyle modification, which includes advice on diet and exercise to improve glycaemic control, reduce insulin resistance and improve cardiovascular fitness. Most people with type 2 diabetes will inevitably require treatment with OHA either due to no symptom relief or persistent poor glycaemic control. The UKPDS confirmed that type 2 diabetes is progressive, resulting in reduced pancreatic beta cell function and increasing insulin resistance. Newly diagnosed patients should be warned from the beginning about the nature of type 2 diabetes to prevent disappointment or feelings of failure when OHA's are prescribed.

Drug selection depends on the patient's weight and severity of glycaemic control or symptoms. Adherence to lifestyle modification and dietary compliance is encouraged.

Biguanides

Metformin is the oral agent of choice particularly for the overweight patients as it may help with weight loss. Its mode of action is to inhibit hepatic glucose output and increase peripheral glucose uptake. Metformin does not increase circulating insulin or cause hypoglycaemia. It should not be used in patients with renal impairment (serum creatinine >150 μmol/l) or with severe heart and liver failure due to the risk of lactic acidosis. A common side-effect is gastrointestinal disturbance and for this reason a low dose should be commenced, for example 500 mg twice daily given with or after food, titrated as necessary. Metformin can be used in combination with sulphonylureas, thiazolidinediones or a long-acting insulin analogue.

Sulphonylureas: gliclazide, glipizide, glimepiride

These OHA's are first-line agents for patients with type 2 diabetes who are particularly thin or who have not been able to tolerate Metformin. They stimulate insulin release by binding to specific receptors on the pancreatic beta cell. They can cause hypoglycaemia and weight gain. A low dose should be prescribed to begin with, which should be taken 20–30 minutes before food, to try and match blood insulin levels with food absorption. Use with caution in patients with hepatic or renal disease. The sulphonylureas available have various duration of action, and can be used in combination with Metformin, thiazolidinediones or a long-acting insulin analogue.

Prandial glucose regulators: nateglinide, repaglinide

Short-acting agents that stimulate insulin secretion and are designed to control post prandial hyperglycaemia. Taken just before each meal, they can cause hypoglycaemia but are often used for patients who have problems with hypoglycaemia, because of their short duration of action.

Thiazolidinediones: rosiglitazone, pioglitazone

The exact mode of action of these agents is not known. They are thought to improve insulin sensitivity and reduce peripheral insulin resistance. A glucose lowering effect is not seen for at least one month after usage has been commenced. They should be taken once a day before or with breakfast, beginning with a low dose and then titrated as necessary. Caution should be taken with patients who have heart failure or liver disease because of the potential for drug interaction with other medications (British National Formulary (BNF), 2003). Both manufacturers recommend liver function tests bimonthly in the first year of treatment, and periodically thereafter. They can be used in combination with Metformin or sulphonylureas, subject to NICE guidance (NICE, 2003c).

HYPOGLYCAEMIA

Hypoglycaemia is feared by people who take insulin therapy and can also be an issue for patients taking a sulphonylurea for the treatment of type 2 diabetes. Education is vital from the outset, regarding the prevention, recognition and treatment of hypoglycaemia. Carrying glucose tablets or sweets and identification is essential advice. Consideration should be given to the timing of meals, eating out, social activities, exercise and alcohol consumption. Glucagon 1 mg injection kits may be offered to the relative or carer for administration in severe hypoglycaemic episodes and could be prescribed by the specialist nurse if included in a CMP.

BLOOD GLUCOSE MONITORING

Blood glucose monitoring is a valuable method of monitoring the effectiveness of therapy and provides information on trends or patterns in blood glucose values that may result in treatment titration or action for example treating a hypoglycaemic event. The value of the results depends on patient participation and compliance with the technique. There are eleven blood glucose meters available, each with different features to compliment the complex needs of individual patients. All now include the reagent strips, a method of quality control, batteries and have reliable customer service. Blood glucose meters can be purchased or obtained at diabetes clinics.

REVIEW

Diabetes is a chronic condition and requires review either annually or periodically, depending on the type of diabetes, level of glycaemic control and the presence of complications. This review can be done by diabetes care teams in primary or secondary care, or as shared care. Annual screening for the complications associated with diabetes includes eye screening, feet examination and urine sampling for albumin creatinine ratio. Blood tests would include glycosylated haemoglobin to assess overall diabetes control and Biochemical profiles for liver and renal function. Lipid profile to assess cholesterol, and triglyceride values, may result in the addition of lipid lowering agents in combination with dietary advice. Monitoring weight is a useful indicator for assessing therapy choices and progress and referral to a dietician for review should be considered.

Diabetic patients are at an increased risk of cardiovascular events (Perry *et al.*, 2003) and blood pressure management is thought to be as important as glycaemic control (UKPDS, 1998). Blood pressure consistently over 140/90 mmHg should be lowered with lifestyle changes, dietary modification and medication to levels below 140/80 mmHg. In 2002, NICE issued guidelines for the management of blood pressure and lipids in people with type 2 diabetes to support the care provided by healthcare professionals to limit or prevent the complications of the disease (NICE, 2002).

References (diabetes)

British Medical Association and the Royal Pharmaceutical Society of Great Britain. (2003). London: British National Formulary.

Diabetes UK (2002). *Diabetes and Pregnancy*. London: Diabetes UK.

DoH (2001a). *National Service Framework for Diabetes: Standards.* London: Department of Health.

DoH (2001b). *National Service Framework for Diabetes.* London: Department of Health.

DoH (2001c). *The Expert Patient. A New Approach to Disease Management for the 21st Century.* London: Department of Health.

DoH (2002a). *Extending Independent Nurse Prescribing within the NHS in England : A Guide for Implementation.* London: The Stationery Office.

DoH (2002b). *National Service Framework. A Practical Aid to Implementation in Primary Care.* London: Department of Health.

European guidelines on cardiovascular disease prevention in clinical practice (2003). *European Heart Journal* **24**: 1601–1610.

NICE (2002). *Guidance on the Management of Blood Pressure and Lipids in Type 2 Diabetes*: Clinical Guidance H.

NICE (2003a). *Guidance on the Use of Patient – Education Models for Diabetes.* Technology Appraisal Guidance No. 60.

NICE (2003b). *Guidance on the Use of Patient – Education Models for Diabetes.* Technology Appraisal Guidance No. 60.

NICE (2003c). *Guidance on the Use of Glitazones for the treatment of Type 2 Diabetes.* Technology Appraisal Guidance No. 63.

Perry CG, Kernohan AFB, Petrie JR (2003). Hypertension in diabetes: what's new, what's true, what's next? *Practical Diabetes International* **20(7)**: 247–254.

Thynne AD, Higgins B, Cummings MH (2003). Choice of insulins, pen devices and blood glucose meters: factors influencing decision making by DSN's in the UK. *Practical Diabetes International* **20(7)**: 237–242.

UK Prospective Diabetes Study Group (1998). Tight blood pressure control and risk of macrovascular and microvascular complications in type 2 diabetes: UKPDS 38. *British Medical Journal* **317**: 703–713.

Chapter 9

Promoting concordance in prescribing interactions: the evidence base and implications for the new generation of prescribers

Sue Latter

INTRODUCTION

The introduction and roll out of nurse prescribing is part of modernising the health service to make it accessible and responsive to patient needs. As greater numbers of professionals begin to exercise their prescribing powers across a wide range of healthcare settings, with an increasing range of medicines, this increases the points of access that patients have to obtaining medicines. However, gaining access to medicines from practitioners is unlikely to improve patients' health *per se*. Increasing access must be combined with a prescribing consultation in which the communication and interaction that occurs enables patients to take their medicines effectively for the benefits of their health.

Using the evidence base for effective prescribing, when effectiveness is measured in terms of potential health benefit, must include not only a consideration of the pharmacological evidence, but also the communication with patients that is required for effective medicine taking. The communication and attitudinal processes that are believed to embody an effective, partnership model of prescribing are known as 'concordance'.

This chapter gives an overview of the evidence base for the concept of concordance, and draws out the implications from research for the new generation of prescribers who wish to practice in the most effective manner possible. It will begin by defining concordance and tracing its history and relationship to the concepts of 'compliance' and 'adherence'. A review of research into both compliance and also concordance is followed by an outline of the reasons why practitioners who are independent (IP)/or supplementary prescribers (SPs) need to incorporate the principles of concordance into their practice. An overview of the skills and competencies that prescribing nurses need in order to adopt concordance in practice will then be presented. This is followed by a section on a review of research that has investigated nurses' and other healthcare professionals' concordance practice; this section will draw conclusions about the extent to which healthcare professionals practice concordance and will also illuminate the factors that are considered to be necessary to put concordance into practice in prescribing interactions.

WHAT IS CONCORDANCE?

The term 'concordance' is used to refer to a partnership approach to interactions about medicines between healthcare professionals and patients. Philosophically and practically, it is used in place of the terms 'compliance' and 'adherence' as goals of medicine interactions, as the latter reflect an inappropriate emphasis on professional dominance and instructing or persuading the patient to comply or adhere to what the healthcare professional perceives to be important in medicine taking. Compliance and adherence also refer to the intended *outcomes* of medicine interactions, whereas concordance is about what happens in the *process* of an interaction, but with important links to effective outcomes of the interaction.

The term 'concordance' was first introduced in 1997 by the Royal Pharamaceutical Society of Great Britain (RPSGB), and has been defined as:

> *a new approach to prescribing and taking medicines, based on partnership. The patient and the healthcare professional participate as partners to reach an agreement on the illness and treatment. Their agreement draws on the experiences, beliefs and wishes of the patient to decide when, how and why to use medicines. Healthcare professionals treat one another as partners and recognise each others' skills to improve the patient's participation*
>
> Medicines Partnership (2003)

From this definition, it can be seen that there is a requirement to share experiences about medicines between the healthcare professional and the patient, and to reach an agreement and work in a co-operative way. Concordance is no different than adopting a partnership approach to other aspects of care and treatment that are provided for patients, but the term itself has come to be used in relation to medicine and prescribing interactions.

The promotion of concordance as the best practice approach within prescribing interactions has arisen for a number of reasons including the fact that there remains a significant clinical and health care problem associated with medicine use, and the evidence base indicates that concordance is an effective way of helping to reduce this problem.

THE PRESCRIBING PROBLEM

Patients do not always take medicines as prescribed, and this phenomenon has been described as 'non-compliance'. Current estimates of non-compliance indicate that this is a prevalent practice: for example, Haynes *et al.* (1996) point out that about half of the medicines prescribed for patients with long-term conditions are not taken as prescribed. Patients can be non-compliant in a number of different ways and it is important for nurses to be aware of these. Vermeire *et al.* (2001) highlight some of the stages and opportunities for non-compliance:

- receiving a prescription, but not having it made up at pharmacy (primary non-compliance),

- taking an incorrect dose,

- taking the medication at the wrong times,

- forgetting one or more doses of the medication,

- stopping the treatment too soon, by ceasing to take the medication sooner than the prescriber recommended or failing to obtain a repeat prescription (secondary non-compliance).

Deliberately or unintentionally not taking medicines as prescribed may have impacts on both patients' health and that of their families or carers and also influences negatively the efficient and effective use of healthcare resources. The origins of this continuing problem are multi-factoral as Marinker and Shaw (2003 p1) point out, 'patients do not comply with medication for several reasons. Non-compliance may be unintentional or involuntary. It may relate to the quality of information given, the impact of the regimen on daily life, the physical or mental incapacity of patients, or their social isolation.'

It is also important to realise that the impact of not taking medicines as intended by the prescriber may be perceived as either positive or negative by patients, and as such needs to be understood within the context of each individual's beliefs and lifestyle. The perceived impact of not taking medicines as prescribed may also differ between the patient and the healthcare professional prescriber. Furthermore, the perceived and actual impact of non-compliant medicine taking may be more or less open to negotiation within a prescribing encounter. For example, a person may chose to take a lower dose of the medicine than has been prescribed because he/she wishes to manage the unpleasant side-effects caused by the medication, and prefers to accommodate the attenuated and incompletely controlled symptoms of the illness than experience side-effects. This example of non-compliance may be mediated within a prescribing encounter if the patient's views and beliefs on current management and medication are sought in an non-judgemental way, understood and perhaps an alternative medication offered with fewer side-effects. Alternatively, another patient may cease to take their prescribed medication before completing the course because they generally hold negative and (scientifically) incorrect views about the medicine in conjunction with the fact that they have become asymptomatic in regard to their illness. Again, the non-compliance may be open to negotiation if the prescriber is able to elicit the patient's views about medicines and negotiate these, in conjunction with providing information about the significance of lack of symptoms.

This begins to suggest that: non-compliance is complex, is best understood individually, may have negative impacts on both the patient's health, and that of their family or carers as well as the efficient and effective use of healthcare resources, and that resolution of these issues demands a partnership approach to interactions in which the patient's views are sought in a non-judgemental manner and understood as a basis for possible negotiation.

EFFECTIVE INTERVENTIONS – THE EVIDENCE BASE

Clearly, the reasons why patients do not take medicines as prescribed are complex. The evidence base for practice in this area is incomplete, but suggests that interventions required to address this issue are also multi-factoral and complex, but that a concordance approach is likely to be one of the most effective strategies that a prescriber can adopt to influence and promote effective medicine taking. An overview of the evidence base for promoting effective medicine interactions is given below.

COMPLIANCE RESEARCH

From the 1970s to the 1990s, research into medicine taking was driven by the professional need to understand and predict non-compliance and to evaluate interventions that promoted compliance. The emphasis was on what needed to be done in order for patients to follow prescriptions as health professionals intended; characteristics of non-compliant patients were sought as well as the best methods of improving compliance. It is perhaps because the research questions driving this field of enquiry were too simplistic, and did not include research into patients' perspectives on the process and influences on medicine taking, that definitive answers to the question of compliance and how to ensure it, were never found. That is to say, working from a professionally defined agenda (compliance) without taking account of patients' perspective is not likely to yield very conclusive results in understanding how to prescribe medicines effectively. Nevertheless, it is useful here to present a summary of what others have distilled from these decades of compliance research, before moving on to research focusing on concordance and its effectiveness.

Both Haynes *et al.*'s (1996) Cochrane review of interventions to promote adherence and Vermeire *et al.*'s (2001) review of research into adherence reach similar conclusions about both what is known in this area and the strength of the evidence base from which this knowledge derives. Haynes *et al.*'s Cochrane review was based on randomised controlled trial research only. The authors concluded that single interventions were unlikely to be effective in promoting adherence and that multiple interventions were required, including, for example, written information and reminders or follow up.

Vermeire *et al.*'s (2001) review includes a broader range of research and other literature on adherence, but also draws similar conclusions. Vermeire *et al.* comment on a range of strategies that have been studied in adherence research, most of which have at least some evidence to support them. These include:

- practical compliance aids such as blister packs, dosage counters and calenders,
- adequate labelling and written information,
- oral information provided by pharmacists,
- educational strategies,
- checking understanding and providing feedback,
- reducing the complexity of the treatment regime,
- encouraging family support.

However, it is important to contextualise these strategies by re-iterating Vermeire *et al.*'s more general conclusions from their review that conclusions about what works are inconsistent across research studies and are also underpinned by research that is often methodologically flawed. In relation to strategies to enhance compliance, Vermeire *et al.* conclude that studies have led to partial and conflicting conclusions and that, to date, there is no evidence that any one method improves compliance better than another.

Similarly, on the causes of 'poor compliance' they conclude: 'to date, none of the suggested explanations has accounted for more than a modest part of observed variations in compliance. Almost 200 different doctor-, patient- and encounter-related variables have been studied but none of them is consistently related to compliance or fully predictive.'

They also comment on the variable quality of research into compliance, the lack of any theoretical framework to test interventions and notable gaps in the research base such as that focusing on patient perspectives and the use of qualitative methods to better understand what promotes adherence.

This review of compliance research highlights that the causes of and solutions to the issue of non-compliance are elusive and unlikely to be discovered through a lens that focuses only on the professionally determined perspective known as compliance. What should nurses and the new generation of prescribers learn from these decades of research? Perhaps it is important to be aware of the repertoire of strategies, such as those outlined above, that have accrued *some* evidence to suggest that they may enhance 'compliance', even if this is incomplete and only partially understood. Nurses prescribing independently or in supplementary mode, may then draw on these strategies selectively and appropriately as part of an individualised approach to their prescribing interactions with patients.

The research review of Vermeire *et al.* (2001) also includes research and other literature on the effectiveness of characteristics of what is now known as concordance, and this evidence is reviewed below.

THE EVIDENCE BASE FOR CONCORDANCE

It is widely advocated that part of the repertoire of interventions necessary for effective medicine taking is a 'partnership approach' to the medicines consultation itself. But what evidence do we have for the effectiveness of this strategy, and how does it compare with the evidence for the other interventions that have been outlined above? In short, the evidence base for recommending a concordance approach to medicine interactions is also incomplete, but research in this area does suggest that concordance produces positive outcomes for patients. The reasons for recommending concordance as the preferred approach to interactions are also practical, ethical and philosophical, as will be outlined below.

Firstly, what is the research evidence that underpins concordance? Both research into the impact of health professionals' communication skills and theoretical models predictive of health behaviour are relevant here. The RPS's (1997) recommendations about concordance are underpinned by the importance of health beliefs in predicting medicine taking as a rationale for adopting concordance as the preferred approach to practice. They suggest that the most salient influences on medicine taking are patients' beliefs about medications and about medicines in general, and these therefore need to be elicited in the prescribing encounter as part of a concordance approach. Certainly, Horne's work (1997) on medicine-related beliefs appears to support such conclusions from the RPS. Vermeire *et al.* (2001) also comment on the place of health beliefs in predicting medicine taking: they highlight, for example, that the Health Belief Model has been helpful in our understanding of compliance.

However, whilst the evidence is suggestive of the importance of health beliefs in predicting medicine-taking behaviour, the elements of most of the health behaviour models have only been partially studied empirically, and, as Vermeire *et al.* (2001) point out: 'there is an immense need for social and psychological research models in order to study patients' attitudes and subjective perceptions ... most of the published explanatory models are only partially satisfactory and hence have been seldom studied experimentally.'

In the absence of definitive research evidence about the importance of patients' health beliefs, it is perhaps important to return to the earlier discussion about the prescribing problem of non-adherence to medicines. This makes clear that the roots often lie within the patient and the extent to which the medicines prescribed are consistent with patients' beliefs and lifestyles. Lack of compliance with prescribed medication is often a rational and intelligent decision on the part of patients that is consistent with their priorities and well being. Therefore, the practical and common sense necessity of exploring these within the prescribing interaction becomes clear – perhaps as a precursor to negotiation or the offer of information or explanation by the healthcare professional. This negotiation between the beliefs and priorities of, on the one hand, the patient, and on the other, the healthcare professional prescribing the medicine, is the essence of concordance. It is a respect for each party's knowledge and experiences that defines the concordance process.

The research evidence for the positive impact of communication skills that are consistent with concordance also point to the need to use this approach in practice. Cox *et al.* (2003) conclude from their review of communication between patients and healthcare professionals about medicine taking that concordance communication, such as encouraging patient participation and listening attentively to patients' views and concerns, may lead to improved outcomes, including enhanced adherence and satisfaction. Vermeire *et al.* (2001) also conclude that 'the literature contains sufficient evidence on the relationship between aspects of communication and the outcomes of patient satisfaction, recall and compliance for positive correlations to be made.'

Similarly, Carter *et al.* (2003) conclude from their review, *A question of choice – compliance in medicine taking*, that 'the available evidence, though incomplete, supports the view that holistic, patient-centred approaches – like concordance (patient–professional partnership in prescribing and medicines management) – are required to address poor compliance.'

The research evidence here does seem to point then to the importance of using communication skills to promote partnership and concordance in practice in pursuit of effective prescribing interactions.

The promotion of concordance is also a reflection of the philosophical shift within policy and practice generally towards greater user involvement and participation in decision-making within clinical encounters. The increasing interest in promoting partnership in healthcare professional: patient interactions is reflected in, for example, the Expert Patient Programme (Department of Health (DoH), 2001), which highlights the need to make use of the expertise and experience of patients in managing their chronic diseases such as asthma, arthritis and diabetes. This programme too is based not only on an ideology of partnership, but also on evidence which indicates that promoting self efficacy and patient ability to take control over managing their own illness is more effective than healthcare professionals trying to do it for them.

Therefore, concordance is advocated as part of the preferred philosophical approach to clinical practice, in addition to the empirical and practical reasons outlined above.

To summarise, the rise in popularity of concordance as an approach to medicine interactions reflects both the evidence base about effective interventions for medicine management, as well as a practical problem of adherence to medicines and a philosophical stance, reflected in key contemporary policy, that places patient participation and partnership at the heart of healthcare, including medicines management.

WHAT ARE THE SKILLS AND KNOWLEDGE REQUIRED TO PRACTICE CONCORDANCE?

A closer examination of the principal components of concordance begins to highlight what knowledge and skills IP and SPs might require in order to put concordance into practice effectively.

The Medicines Partnership (2003) outlines three essential components of concordance:

1. *Patients have enough knowledge to participate as partners*: This involves offering patients information about medicines that is clear, accurate, accessible, sufficiently detailed and tailored to individual needs.

2. *Prescribing consultations involve patients as partners*: This means that patients are invited to talk openly about their priorities, preferences and concerns about medicine taking and treatment. Professionals explain the rationale for, and the characteristics of the proposed treatment. Patients and health professionals jointly agree on a course of treatment that reconciles as far as possible the professional's recommendations and the patient's preferences. The patient's and the professional's understanding of what has been agreed is checked, as well as the patient's ability to follow the agreed treatment.

3. *Patients are supported in taking their medicines*: This requires that all opportunities be taken to discuss medicines issues, that healthcare professionals share medicines information effectively with one another. It also means that medications are reviewed regularly, with patients' participation and that practical difficulties in taking medicines are addressed.

This suggests that skills in information giving and explanations about medicines, as well as using communication skills to elicit patient perspectives are indicated.

The National Prescribing Centre's (NPCs) (2003) outline of prescribing competencies also reflects the importance of concordance as the preferred method of communication within prescribing consultations, and highlights skills and knowledge similar to those identified by Medicines Partnership (2003) above. For example, the NPC standard on *communicating with patients* identifies that the prescriber:

- establishes a relationship based on trust and mutual respect,

- sees patients as partners in the consultation,

- applies the principles of concordance.

And competencies to achieve this include:

- listening to patient's beliefs and expectations,

- dealing sensitively with the patient's emotions and concerns,

- helping patients to make informed choices,

- offering explanations and rationales for treatment options,

- negotiating outcomes of consultations that both prescriber and patient are satisfied with,

- giving clear instructions to patients about their medication,

- checking the patient's understanding of and commitment to treatment.

This again suggests that what is required are skills in information giving, and using communication skills such as open questions, listening skills and picking up on cues to encourage patients to share their agenda, and their beliefs and expectations about medicines (see Chapter 3 for further information on consultation skills and decision-making).

Such skills are important, but need to be used in conjunction with the prescriber's reflection on attitudes and beliefs about the purpose of the interaction, i.e. that what is required is for the healthcare professional to use skills that facilitate the overall goal of supporting patients and using opportunities to contribute to the decisions that they currently make about medication – decisions that fit with the patient's own beliefs and personal circumstances.

It is also important to highlight that the skills and competencies of concordance will also often be used by nurses within the context of an existing or on-going relationship with a patient. This pattern of contact may well be different to that available to other prescribers such as doctors and pharmacists, and this may therefore represent an opportunity for nurses to improve on the often poor communication that has characterised doctors' prescribing interactions in the past, as demonstrated for example in Cox *et al.*'s (2003) systematic review (see below). Not only do nurses often have on-going relationships with their patients, they are also often valued by patients specifically for professional and personal characteristics such as approachability and accessibility. This fact has also been highlighted in early evaluations of nurse prescribing: Latter and Courtenay's (2004) review of literature on the effectiveness of nurse prescribing found that one of the key positive elements to emerge from the first wave of nurse prescribing in the UK was the value that patients placed on their relationship with their prescribing nurse. Nurses therefore need to exploit this in the interests of effective medicine management by ensuring that they are building on their relationships with patients where possible and are using the skills and competencies of concordance in the context of this valued relationship.

The skills and competencies outlined above also make it clear that concordance involves effective communication between members of the healthcare team and regular review of prescribed medicines, a requirement that is consistent with Government recommendations on supplementary prescribing.

Experienced nurses reading this will perhaps consider that they already do this, that they have a holistic, partnership approach to interactions, including those focused on medicines, as well as the communication skills required to put this approach into practice operationally. Often these principles and skills are perceived as 'second nature' to nurses and something that they have simply acquired as part of their clinical experience. However, the majority of research investigating nurses' and other healthcare professionals' approach to medicines interactions strongly points to the conclusion that their interactions fall short of demonstrating concordance in practice. A review of this research and its implications for IP and SPs is given below.

CONCORDANCE – WHAT ARE HEALTHCARE PROFESSIONALS DOING IN PRACTICE?

Prior to the emergence of concordance as a concept and as an ideal for practice, research in the realm of prescribing and medicines management focused on describing and evaluating patient compliance and adherence to medicines prescribed by doctors. Interventions to promote compliance were also evaluated, often by using randomised controlled trials, although, as highlighted above, overall conclusions about the most effective interventions have remained elusive.

More recently, there have been a small number of studies that have looked specifically at the processes nurses employ within medicine interactions, or the extent to which the principles of concordance are being put into practice operationally. A systematic review of research into communication between patients and healthcare professionals about medicine taking and prescribing has also recently become available (Cox et al., 2003). Whilst research into concordance in practice remains scarce to date, a review of the available evidence begins to shed light on current practice and enables some implications for prescribing nurses to be drawn from this.

The aim of the systematic review undertaken by Cox et al. (2003) was to identify and summarise research on two-way communication between patients and healthcare professionals in order to inform the model of concordance. The review focused on 134 qualitative and quantitative studies published between 1991 and 2000 and included both intervention and non-intervention studies that spanned a variety of countries. Most of the studies examined elements of what is now known as concordance, even if the original studies did not define them as such – for example, research into 'encouraging patients to ask questions about medicines' and 'involving patients in discussions about medicines' is reviewed. Unsurprisingly, the majority of studies have focused on doctors' communication about medicines, with a minority also describing pharmacist and patient communication behaviours. Comparatively few studies in the review focus on nurses, and this is perhaps not surprising given the relatively recent emergence of nurses internationally into the prescribing arena. However, valuable insights and lessons for nurses can be drawn from previous research into doctor and pharmacist communication behaviours with patients about their medicines.

From their review Cox *et al.* (2003) conclude that 'Much of the research indicated that communication between patients and professionals retains the asymmetry typical of paternalistic healthcare professional-patient interactions. ... Therefore the evidence examined in this review suggests that it is unlikely that concordance is taking place.'

The authors do however note that there was evidence that it was possible to move towards a concordant approach in practice if certain pre-conditions were in place such as doctors encouraging patient participation and listening attentively to their concerns. They also note that where some degree of concordance had taken place in practice, positive outcomes were noted, such as improved satisfaction and adherence.

This therefore adds weight to the argument that nurses and other healthcare professionals should be striving for concordance in practice. The conclusions also point to the fact that healthcare professionals have some way to go to achieve it.

A more detailed analysis of Cox *et al.*'s review is beyond the scope of this chapter, but, in addition to the above overall conclusions, the review also highlights that patient preferences for participation and partnership in interactions and decision-making are complex and dynamic. As with the research into the more general concept of patient participation, the research in Cox *et al.*'s review indicates that patients vary in the extent to which they wish to, for example engage in discussion about medicines and share decisions about medicine management. It is likely that these preferences may be at least partly bound up with previous experiences and expectations about roles and relationships in healthcare interactions (Latter *et al.*, 2000). That is, if a patient has not experienced a two-way communication process with a healthcare professional, then he/she may not know how empowered he/she would feel if given the opportunity to become involved.

Two recent studies focusing specifically on the role and practice of nurses and aspects of medicines management draw similar conclusions to Cox *et al.*'s (2003) review, and also help shed further detail on how nurses are practising and what is required in order to progress towards a more concordant approach in practice.

Latter *et al.*'s (2000) study into nurses' role in medication education found that nurses across a range of clinical settings were generally found to limit their role in patient medication education to simple information about the name of the drug, its purpose and time of administration. There was little patient involvement in decisions about medication and little evidence to suggest that nurses were using the skills of concordance in practice, or were indeed aware of the evidence base about what should be used in practice. Patients also had relatively low expectations about the degree of involvement that they would have liked in these medication interactions – although there was some evidence from a minority of patients, and also carers, that they would have liked greater involvement and/or information about medicines, suggesting, as highlighted above, that preferences for involvement and information are likely to vary from patient to patient and should be explored and assessed thoroughly on an individualised basis. This study also identified influences, both positive and negative, that impacted on nurses' ability to interact with patients about medication in a manner consistent with the principles of concordance. Patients' preferences for a low level of detail about their medication were cited by nurses as inhibitory, as well as lack of time available and high workload. On the other hand, interactions were more sophisticated where the organisation of care facilitated a good nurse–client relationship and where the clinical area was nurse-led rather than care decisions determined by medical or organisational priorities.

Similar findings emerged from Rycroft-Malone's (2002) study, which focused specifically on patient participation in nurse–patient interactions about medication using a variety of qualitative methods, including conversational analysis as a data analysis technique. She found that a range of conversational strategies was employed by nurses to initiate and control conversations and by doing so inhibited patients' participation. Predominantly, nurses did not encourage patients to take part in concordance type interactions, by, for example, assessing health beliefs and facilitating participation in decision-making. Rycroft-Malone did however find that there was a range in the extent to which the nurses in her study facilitated participation, and the extent to which they were able to do this was dependent on a number of factors. These were:

- power,
- nurses' communication style,
- knowledge, skills and experience,
- patients' age, acuity of illness and level of knowledge,
- organisation and philosophy of care.

Where nurses had more training in communication skills, as well as more extensive clinical experience and qualifications, their interactions exhibited greater characteristics of participation, in the manner of concordance. Similar to Latter et al., (2000), she found that participation and concordance were also facilitated in settings where the philosophy and organisation of care emphasised patient-centeredness, and continuity of care and relationship building. Rycroft-Malone also found however, that the influence of power, both of the institution in which nurses in her study worked and the personal power of nurses themselves, was an all pervading influence and mitigating factor against promoting patient participation in medication encounters. A more detailed review of this study is beyond the scope of this chapter, but the findings do both underline the fact that evidence suggests concordance is not yet a feature of practice and it also begins to identify some of the factors that prescribing nurses may need to attend to if they are to enact concordance and patient participation in practice. Both Latter et al.'s (2000) and Rycroft-Malone's (2002) study indicate that where good nurse–patient relationships are fostered, concordance may be enhanced. This relationship building may be a function of both training in communication skills, and also practising in settings where the organisation of care facilitates this.

The research to date cited above does however focus predominantly on non-nurses (Cox *et al.*, 2003), or nurses who were administering medicines rather than prescribing them, often to patients who were acutely ill (Latter *et al.*, 2000; Rycroft-Malone, 2002). It is to be hoped that both the educational preparation for independent and supplementary prescribing, as well as the settings in which these prescribers work, will enable nurses to use their skills and clinical experience to begin to apply the principles of concordance in practice.

CONCLUSION

In this chapter, the meaning of concordance has been explored, together with an examination of the evidence base for its effectiveness in practice. Concordance has been compared with the traditional approach of compliance in medicine taking, and the evidence base for the latter has been shown to be inadequate in a number of respects. Knowledge and skills needed to enact concordance in practice have been outlined. Whilst these may *appear* to be skills that nurses are familiar with, a warning against complacency is given by an examination of the research in this area to date – which suggests that concordance is not yet a feature of nurses' medicine interactions with patients.

Further research is required, encompassing both descriptive research into what prescribing nurses are doing in practice, and also research that will contribute to the existing evidence base about the effectiveness of concordance approaches in practice.

Concordance is advocated as a key competency for nurses and other health professionals who are now the new generation of prescribers. To move towards its use in practice is likely to maximise the true potential that the extension of prescribing powers represents, by enhancing not only patient access to the prescription of medicines, but also their access to medicine encounters that will truly enhance their ability to manage their medicines for the benefit of their health and well being.

References

Carter S, Taylor D, Levenson R (2003). *A Question of Choice – Compliance in Medicine Taking.* London: Medicines Partnership.

Cox K, Stevenson F, Britten N, Dundar Y (2003). *A Systematic Review of Communication between Patients and Healthcare Professionals about Medicine-taking and Prescribing.* London: Guys Kings and St Thomas Concordance Unit.

Department of Health (2001). *The Expert Patient Programme.* London: Department of Health.

Haynes RB, McKibbon KA, Kanani R, Brouwers MC, Oliver T (1997). *Interventions to Assist Patients to Follow Prescriptions for Medications* Issue 2. Oxford: Cochrane Library.

Horne R (1997). Representations of medication and treatment: advances in theory and measurement. In: *Perceptions of Health and Illness: Current Research and Applications* (Petrie, R and Weinman, J). London: Harwood Academic. pp. 155–188.

Latter S, Courtenay M (2004). Effectiveness of nurse prescribing: a review of the literature. *Journal of Clinical Nursing* **13**: 26–32.

Latter S, Yerrell P, Rycroft-Malone J, Shaw D (2000). *Nursing and Medication Education; Concept Analysis Research for Curriculum and Practice Development. Research Reports Series No 15.* London: English National Board for Nursing, Midwifery and Health Visiting.

Marinker M, Shaw J (2003). Not to be taken as directed: putting concordance for taking medicines into practice. *British Medical Journal* **326**: 348–349.

Medicines Partnership (2003). *Project Evaluation Toolkit.* London: Medicines Partnership.

National Prescribing Centre (2003). *An Outline Framework to Help Nurse Prescribers.* Liverpool: NHS National Prescribing Centre.

Royal Pharmaceutical Society of Great Britain (1997). *From Compliance to Concordance: Achieving Shared Goals in Medicine-taking.* London: The Royal Pharmaceutical Society of Great Britian.

Rycroft-Malone J (2002). *Patient Participation in Nurse-patient Interactions About Medication.* Unpublished PhD thesis, School of Nursing and Midwifery University of Southampton.

Vermeire E, Hearnshaw H, Van Royen P, Denekens J (2001). Patient adherence to treatment: three decades of research. A comprehensive review. *Journal of Clinical Pharmacy and Therapeutics* **26**: 331–342.

Chapter 10

Evidence-based prescribing

Trudy Granby and Stephen R Chapman

INTRODUCTION

According to Sackett *et al.* (1996) evidence-based healthcare is:

> *judiciously and conscientiously applying the best evidence to prevent, detect and treat disorders*

This is an ambitious statement, as the barriers to disseminating and applying evidence are both numerous and multifaceted.

The discipline of evidence-based medicine (EBM) is relatively new to nurses; traditionally they have based their clinical decisions on a combination of experience, observation, opinion, published material and personal research (Trinder and Reynolds, 2000). The introduction of clinical governance, which emphasises accountability, quality and efficiency, has challenged this approach and it is no longer acceptable to base clinical decisions on personal opinion. Decision-making must be evidence-based.

Prescribing is only one stage in making a rational treatment decision. Other stages include drawing on individual clinical expertise, taking account of patient choice and considering available resources. This needs to follow a 'stepwise' approach, starting with defining the patient's problem, which requires specific clinical skills and expertise, including undertaking a detailed history and physical examination, interpreting test results etc. In some circumstances, treatment may be initiated before a firm diagnosis has been made. In this situation, the clinician has to draw upon the best information available at the time and their knowledge of the patient.

It is essential that the patient is involved in making the treatment decisions. The patient's beliefs, expectations and preferences should be identified and acknowledged alongside existing clinical evidence. If a treatment is unacceptable to a patient, they are unlikely to adhere to the regime.

Evidence-based clinical practice is an approach to decision-making. It is about considering, and then applying, the best evidence available when deciding how to treat an individual patient, groups of patients, or populations (Gray, 1997).

It is a structured process and requires the practitioner to be able to:

- Recognise and understand certain criteria, such as safety, effectiveness and efficacy.

- Access evidence and assess its quality.

- Recognise whether the results can be generalised and/or can be applied to the individual, group or population.

This chapter provides a brief insight into some of the issues surrounding evidence-based prescribing including clinical and cost-effectiveness, hierarchy of evidence, recognising the benefits or harm of a treatment, and concordance.

SOME FACTS AND FIGURES

In England during 2002, drugs used to treat chronic conditions such as cardiovascular disease, conditions of the central nervous system, respiratory disease and endocrine disorders accounted for around 60.5% of the total items dispensed from National Health Services (NHS) prescriptions in the community (Department of Health (DoH), 2003a).

Prescribing, supplying and administering medicines is now probably the most common healthcare intervention. In England, during 2002, 617 million items were dispensed from NHS prescriptions in the community, 87.5% of which were free to patients, at a net ingredient cost £6847 million. On average, 12.5 items were dispensed per head of population. (DoH, 2003a). To give a comparison, around 104 million more items were dispensed during 2002 than during 1998, at an increased net ingredient cost of around £2146 million (DoH, 2003b)

In the acute healthcare sector, during 1999/2000, medicines accounted for over £1.5 billion spent by NHS hospitals (which represents around 4.6% of their overall costs). Around £90 million worth of medicines are taken into hospitals every year by patients – most of these are destroyed. 7000 individual doses of medication are administered in a 'typical' hospital every day and administration of medicines takes up approximately 40% of nurses' time (Audit Commission, 2001).

It could be assumed that this massive spending on medicines has resulted in an improvement in the health of the population. Although most patients do benefit from the medicines they are prescribed, this is not always the case; 50% of patients with chronic conditions fail to take their medication as prescribed (DoH, 2000a). Since the introduction of the Yellow Card Scheme in 1964 more than 40,000 suspected adverse reactions to drugs have been reported to the Committee on Safety of Medicines (CSM)/Medicines and Healthcare products Regulatory Agency (MHRA). Around 17% of older inpatients, experience an adverse drug reaction (Audit Commission, 2001) and medication errors cost the NHS around £500 million each year in additional inpatient days. Furthermore, around 25% of clinical negligence cases stem from hospital medication errors (DoH, 2000b).

HOW CAN WE IMPROVE THINGS?

The main focus of the NHS reforms (DoH, 2000c) is to improve the quality of care received by patients by increased access to the services required and the medicines required to treat their illness. One way in which this can be achieved is to extend the roles of some healthcare professionals enabling them to prescribe, supply and administer medicines. If prescribing is to be effective, the practitioner must be able to:

- Identify the problem in terms of the patient's (or population's) needs and the ultimate goal of any treatment.

- Break the problem down into more explicit questions, such as 'What are the treatment options? How well do they work? What are the resource implications?'.

- Check the evidence.

In order to do this, the following must be considered:

HOW EFFECTIVE ARE THE TREATMENT OPTIONS?

To answer the above, two issues must be considered – *efficacy and clinical-effectiveness*. They are quite different.

Efficacy is when a drug is proven to have a pharmacological effect greater than a placebo. This does not necessarily translate into improved clinical outcome. Clinical-effectiveness is when that efficacy results in a proven clinical outcome. For instance, if drug A lowers blood pressure by 2 mmHg it has proven clinical efficacy, and could, in theory get a licence. If, however, using drug A to lower blood pressure by 2 mmHg has no effect on the desired outcome (i.e. it does not have any effect on stroke prevention) then it is not clinically effective.

This is an important differentiation. A drug can be efficacious, and have a licence, but may not be the drug of choice when clinical outcome (i.e. effectiveness) is considered. In other words, just because it has a licence it is not necessarily the optimal drug.

IS THE DRUG COST-EFFECTIVE?

In a publicly-funded, cash-limited health economy such as a Primary Care Trust (PCT) making sure that a drug represents value for money is as much a part of evidence-based prescribing as clinical-effectiveness. It is particularly important to rationalise one's thinking around *marginal benefit*.

This is best illustrated by the following example, outlined in Box 1, of two hypothetical drugs used to treat the common cold – Drug A and Drug B.

Box 1 An illustration of marginal costs and benefits

Drug A cures colds completely in 90% of cases
Drug B cures colds completely in 80% of cases
Drug A costs £10
Drug B costs £5
You have £1000 to treat patients in your PCT
Drug A treats £1000/10 × 90% = 90 patients
Drug B treats £1000/5 × 80% = 160 patients

In this example, you can treat almost twice the number of patients to cure by using a less effective drug. If, however, you had a cold, and you could afford it, you may prefer to pay the extra £5 to cure your cold. Thus you are applying different values when using public money – this tension exists in making all prescribing decisions – having to balance the needs of the individual against the needs of the population.

This active dynamic is illustrated in an article by Barber (1995). He represents this diagrammatically, (Figure 10.1), adding the dimension of patient choice to Parish's (1973, cited in Barber, 1995) original definition of appropriateness, safety, effectiveness, and cost.

Health economies and organisations such as The National Institute of Clinical Excellence (NICE) that seek to balance costs and benefits, use health economic modelling. These models are often complex and sophisticated. Whilst prescribers do not need a detailed knowledge of health economics, it does help to have a basic understanding of the key terms.

In the simplest form, if two drugs have the same clinical effect, then it makes sense to prescribe the cheapest alternative – this is known as *cost-minimisation*.

Cost-effective analysis is one method by which the cost of treatment can be compared with expected outcome, for example reduction in blood pressure. Effectiveness is measured in natural units, such as drop in millimetres of mercury.

Cost-benefit analysis takes this a stage further by allocating a cost to the differences in these natural units. The conventional way of carrying out cost-effectiveness analysis involves considering additional costs over and above the cost of the medicine. These include direct costs (the cost of the medicine, staff time involved in carrying out the therapy, equipment required to do this and any costs to the patient e.g. transport to clinics); indirect costs (how time spent by staff could have been otherwise used) and intangible costs (such as pain and adverse effects) (Phillips and Thompson, 1997).

For example, in a hospital, the intravenous (IV) anaesthetic propofol is more expensive per unit than conventional general anaesthetic, which means that the direct costs are higher. However, using propofol means that patients have fewer side-effects and recover more quickly from the effects of the anaesthetic, which speeds up discharge from hospital. This, in turn, results in more surgical procedures

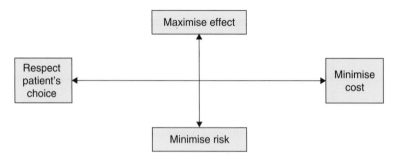

Figure 10.1   Aims of good prescribing – and their commonest conflicts (from Barber, 1995)

being performed as day cases, thus avoiding the 'hotel costs' of overnight accommodation in hospital. Avoiding these direct costs makes propofol more cost-effective. Health economic studies need to be examined as carefully as clinical trials and should be critically appraised before rushing to conclusions – Drummond *et al.*'s paper and that of the evidence-based medicine working group give an excellent guide to key points to check (Drummond, 1997; O'Brien, 1997). There is also an easy-to-read, light-hearted look at a 'crooks guide' on how pharmacoeconomic studies are designed to ensure drugs look cost-effective in the book *Pharmacoeconomics* (Wally *et al.*, 2004).

CHECKING THE EVIDENCE

The evidence available to support prescribing decisions can be derived from a number of sources:

- published evidence,
- personal experience,
- reasoning and intuition,
- colleagues and peers,
- promotional material.

If an effective prescribing decision is to be made, attention to the published evidence is crucial. Published evidence varies in terms of quality and credibility. Studies can therefore be ranked according to a 'hierarchy of evidence' (Table 10.1).

Systematic reviews and/or meta-analysis

Good quality systematic reviews provide the best indication of the effects of an intervention. These reviews use a robust, formalised process to summarise available research evidence (Egger *et al.*, 2001). By asking a number of therapeutic questions, for example the intention of the therapy, the patient group, and the outcome of the intervention, this process identifies those studies that warrant inclusion in the review. The results of studies reviewed are then combined (using meta-analysis) to assess the effectiveness of the intervention. Issues such as the quality of the

Table 10.1　Hierarchy of evidence (Jones, 2002)

I	Systematic reviews and meta-analysis
II	Randomised controlled double blind trials
III	Cohort studies
IV	Case control studies
V	Cross sectional surveys
VI	Case series
VII	Case reports

studies included and the possibility and likely impact of bias and chance are discussed to help contextualise the review.

Systematic reviews are often published in leading journals and can also be accessed via a range of websites (Table 10.2). The Cochrane website is a good independent source for such reviews.

Meta-analysis   is a technique used to combine study findings. This form of analysis is most frequently used to assess the effectiveness of a therapeutic intervention by combing data of two or more randomised controlled trials. The findings of trials involving large numbers are generally more reliable. Combining the results in this

Table 10.2   Some sources of information available from the Internet

Peer-reviewed journals	
Annals of Internal Medicine	www.annals.org
British Medical Journal (BMJ)	www.bmj.com
Journal of the American Medical Association (JAMA)	www.jama.ama-assn.org
New England Journal of Medicine	www.nejm.org
The Lancet	www.thelancet.com
Systematic reviews and digests of reviews	
Aggressive research intelligence facility (ARIF)	http://www.bham.ac.uk/arif
Bandolier	www.jr2.ox.ac.uk/bandolier
Clinical evidence	www.clinicalevidence.com
Cochrane library	www.nelh.nhs.uk/cochrane.asp
Database of abstracts of reviews of effectiveness (DARE)	www.york.ac.uk/inst/crd/darehp.htm
Drugs and therapeutics bulletin	www.dtb.org.uk/dtb/index.html
Effective healthcare bulletins	www.york.ac.uk/inst/crd/ehcb.htm
Effectiveness matters	www.york.ac.uk/inst/crd/em.htm
Evidence-based medicine	ebm.bmjjournals.com/
Health technology assessment	www.york.ac.uk/inst/crd/htahp.htm
MeReC bulletins, briefings and extras	www.npc.co.uk
NHS centre for reviews and dissemination reports	www.york.ac.uk/inst/crd/crdrep.htm
NHS economic evaluation database (NHS EED)	www.york.ac.uk/inst/crd/nhsdhp.htm

Research in progress	
National research register	www.doh.gov.uk/research/nrr.htm
Guidance	
eGuidelines	www.eguidelines.co.uk
Midland therapeutic review and advisory committee (MTRAC)	www.keele.ac.uk/depts/mm/MTRAC/
National institute for clinical excellence	www.nice.org.uk
Prodigy	www.prodigy.nhs.uk
Scottish intercollegiate guidelines network (SIGN)	www.sign.ac.uk/
Other resources	
British National formulary	www.bnf.org
Centre for evidence-based medicine	www.cebm.net/
DrugInfoZone	www.druginfozone.org
Electronic medicines compendium	emc.medicines.org.uk
Medicines partnership	www.medicines-partnership.org
National electronic library for health	www.nelh.nhs.uk
National prescribing centre	www.npc.co.uk
National Service Frameworks	www.doh.gov.uk/nsf/nsfhome.htm
Netting the evidence	www.nettingtheevidence.org.uk
NPC Current awareness bulletin (eCAB)	www.npc.co.uk/ecab/ecab.jsp
Nurse prescriber	www.nurse-prescriber.co.uk
UK Medicines information	www.ukmi.nhs.uk
Virtual health network	www.vhn.net

way provides an estimate of the effects of a particular intervention. However, it must be remembered that any meta-analysis is dependent on the quality of the individual studies. With this in mind, prescribers need to be able to appraise studies and interpret the findings for themselves or, alternatively, check with independent reviews such as Cochrane.

Randomised controlled trials   are normally used to assess the effects of a particular drug. Typically, two groups are studied: one group receives the intervention, whilst the other group acts as the control. Patients are allocated to study groups randomly by a process analogous to 'flipping a coin' to avoid bias. This type of study can be developed further by setting up systems to ensure that neither the researcher nor the patient is aware of who is receiving the intervention. This is known as 'double-blinding.'

Cohort studies   are often used to find out what causes a particular disease. Subjects with a specific disease, or who have certain characteristics, are identified and followed up over a period of time to monitor progress and/or detect complications. For instance, the Framingham study has charted the progress of heart disease, stroke and other conditions in a cohort of American men over 50 years. (www.framingham.com/heart). Cohort studies are often done retrospectively from large databases, such as the General Practice Research database, which have historical data.

Case control studies   examine the causes of a disease. In these studies, a group of patients with a particular disease are compared to a group with similar characteristics (such as age, sex, and concurrent medical conditions) but who do not have the disease. Case control studies compare histories of those in the group to identify any exposure to possible causal factors.

Cross sectional surveys   measure the frequency of a disease or risk factor in a defined group, at a given time. These surveys can be used to determine the prevalence of a condition.

Case reports   are descriptive, anecdotal reports of the medical history of one patient. A *case series* is a collection of similar reports. As there is no control group, case reports and case series are not statistically valid. However, they are useful in alerting others of rare occurrences or the emergence of 'new' diseases.

RECOGNISING THE BENEFITS OR HARMS OF A TREATMENT

In order to decide whether a drug should be prescribed, it is useful to know whether intervening with that drug in an experimental group produced a different effect to intervening with a placebo (i.e. an identical looking tablet or capsule with no active ingredient) in a control group. The results of such trials allow us to estimate the probability of a greater benefit, and/or, what are the risks of harmful outcomes such as side-effects. Benefits and harms are presented in a number of ways, which can affect how they are perceived (Bucher *et al.*, 1994). It is therefore important to have an understanding of what these terms mean, as well as the principles underpinning them.

Results are often presented in terms of reducing risk, either as absolute risk reduction (ARR) or relative risk reduction (RRR). Reporting RRR, tends to show an increased positive effect. Absolute and relative risks are sometimes reported within the same paper. It is important to have an understanding of the differences between the two.

Absolute risk

The absolute risk is the chance of developing a condition, for example the risk of contracting an infection may be 1 in 100,000.

Relative risk

The relative risk is the chance of developing a condition when a factor is present, divided by the risk of developing the condition when that factor is absent. For instance, if 20 out of a 100 patients develop a skin rash when taking a drug, whereas only 5 out of a 100 get a skin rash when taking a placebo, the relative risk is 20/100 divided by 5/100, which is 4. In other words, the risk of developing a rash when taking that drug is four times greater than when not taking the drug.

Caution needs to be taken when examining at relative risk, as it takes no account of background incidence. It should, therefore, always be considered in the context of absolute risk. For example, if the absolute risk of infection is 1 in 100,000, and the relative risk is 2, the risk increases to 2 in 100,000, which is still very low. However, if the absolute risk of infection is 1 in 5, and the relative risk is 2, the risk increases by 2 in 5 – an increase of 20%, which would probably be unacceptable.

Absolute risk reduction

ARR is the absolute amount by which an intervention can reduce the absolute risk. This is calculated as:

$$ARR = \text{(event rate in the control group} - \text{event rate in the intervention group)} \times 100$$

Sackett (2000)

To illustrate this, suppose 2000 people received Drug X (*the intervention group*) and 2000 people received a placebo – *the control group.* The *intention* is to prevent death.

In the intervention group, 360 people died making the event rate 360/2000. In the control group, 500 people died, making the event rate 500/2000.

So, applying the above calculation, the ARR is:

$$\frac{(500 - 360)}{2000} \times 100, \quad \text{i.e.} \quad \frac{140}{2000} \times 100,$$

a reduction in the death rate of 7%.

Relative risk reduction

RRR reports how much a risk is reduced by an intervention as a comparative percentage of the control. This is calculated by dividing the difference between the rate of events in the control and intervention groups by the rate of events in the control group. So, if we relate back to the example used to calculate the ARR, the RRR is:

$$\frac{(360/2000) - (500/2000)}{500/2000},$$

i.e. $\frac{0.07}{0.25}$, a reduction in death rate of 28%.

Number needed to treat

This is probably the most useful way of expressing results as it tells the prescriber how many patients with a given condition they need to treat with a particular intervention before one additional patient benefits. To use Moore and McQuay's (1997) example, let us suppose that 100 people are given an analgesic. Of these, 70 people have their pain relieved within 2 hours. However, when these same 100 people are given a placebo instead of the analgesia, only 20 have their pain relieved within 2 hours. We can assume that the pain was relieved by the analgesia in 50 (70 – 20) cases. This is an ARRs of (70/100 – 20/100) i.e. 0.5.

The number needed to treat (NNT) is calculated by dividing 1 by the ARR, i.e. 1/(control event rate − experimental event rate), in this case 1/0.5, which gives an NNT of 2. This means that two people have to take the analgesic for one of them to obtain relief as a result of taking that analgesic. This is a very low NNT, which means it is an optimal treatment. Although there is no cut off point, once NNTs go over 100 (i.e. over 100 patients have to be treated by a drug for one patient to benefit), prescribers should be more circumspect.

Odds ratios

The odds of an event happening are calculated by taking the number of times something happens and dividing that by the number of times it does not happen. For example, let us say that for every 100 people buying a raffle ticket, 26 win something (the event happens) and 74 do not (the event does not happen). To work out the odds of winning, 26 is divided by 74, making the chance of winning 0.35, i.e. 35%. Any number over 1 means that the chances of winning are good, anything below 1 means that the chances of winning are unlikely.

However, knowing the odds is not enough when deciding whether a drug intervention is effective – this involves knowing whether there is a difference between the odds of something happening to the group receiving a particular intervention, and the control group who do not receive the intervention. This is known as the *odds ratio*, which is calculated by dividing the odds in the treatment group with the odds in the control group.

For example, Drug A, is believed to cure the common cold within 24 hours of the first symptoms appearing. It is given to 100 people and works in 60 cases. Therefore, the odds of this happening in this group are 60/40, which is 1.5. Placebo A is given to another 100 people with the same symptoms. This time 20 people recover in 24 hours, making the odds 20/80, which is 0.25. So, the odds ratio between the two groups is 1.5/0.25, i.e. 6.

As 6 is a much higher number than 1, the odds ratio suggests that drug A is effective and thus worth prescribing. To explain this a little further, if 60 or more people from the placebo group had recovered, the odds ratio would have been 1 or less. This would have shown that the drug had an effect equivalent to, or less than a placebo, and would not be worth prescribing.

Obviously, this is a very simplistic example. In reality, calculating event rates, reported as odds ratios, is not that easy and some would argue against describing the effects of treatments in this way. However, odds ratios are frequently used. This is possibly because they provide a way of presenting benefit (or harm) within a wide range of values: zero to infinity.

Further examples of risk reductions, odds ratios etc are given in Trisha Greenhalgh's book *How to read a paper: the basics of evidence based medicine* (2002).

GUIDELINES

The increase in the amount of available information has, paradoxically, increased the risk of unacceptable variations in the way certain conditions are managed. In order to manage this risk, organisations have produced guidelines (at both national and local levels) to help standardise best practice. Providing these guidelines are robust, reliable, and properly implemented, they are really useful when making prescribing decisions and should improve healthcare by reducing the variations. Applying guidelines to individuals still requires some degree of judgement, as no recommendation can take into account the many varied circumstances of an individual.

Guidelines are used in a range of ways to promote effective and efficient care. Locally developed guidelines should encompass valid, national guidelines, such as NICE Guidance, and should be prioritised to address local need. Some sources of guidelines are listed in the table at the end of this chapter.

FINDING THE EVIDENCE

Keeping up to date with the amount of evidence can be very daunting. In order to make good use of the often limited time available, it should help to know how to keep up to date by knowing which journals should be used and where to find independent reviews of the evidence.

The internet possibly offers the easiest, and most effective route to keeping up to date, and many websites operate an E-mail alert service. Some of these websites are password protected and require a subscription to access full text. However, they do usually allow access to abstracts. The Internet is not without its hazards as anyone can post information on it. Using a standard search engine to look for information may lead to sponsored sites, which may carry an element of bias, or have incomplete information. With this is mind, it is advisable to always check who sponsors the site and ideally restrict your searches to the sites we have listed in Table 10.2.

WILL THE PATIENT FOLLOW THE TREATMENT?

Regardless of the evidence, a medicine can only be effective if the patient follows the treatment regime. There are many, often complicated reasons why a patient fails to do this. In some cases this may be related to the cost of 'cashing in' the prescription (Jones and Britten, 1998). But even when patients have access to their medicine, they do not always follow the prescribers' instructions. This may reflect the clinicians' approach to consultation (see Chapter 3), whereby the patient does not have the opportunity to discuss any concerns (Barry et al., 2000). Indeed, how the consultation is conducted is a cornerstone to the concept of concordance, which is based on the prescriber and patient working together, as equals, to form a 'concord', i.e. a contract or, if you prefer, a therapeutic alliance. The aim of this therapeutic alliance is to create a situation whereby the patient feels able to share the decision-making around the management of their condition, including which medicines are prescribed (Royal Pharmaceutical Society of Great Britain (RPSGB), 1998).

To help make this happen, the prescriber must ensure that the patient has an understanding of their condition and is aware of all of the treatment options, including the associated risks and benefits. This approach is quite the opposite to the prescriber dominated, paternalistic approach associated with compliance whereby the prescriber makes these decisions and instructs the patient on what they should do.

Concordance may present the prescriber with some challenges. By increasing the patient's knowledge about treatment options and inviting them to make decisions about which treatment they would prefer, the patient may not choose what the prescriber considers to be the best option. Furthermore, there may be times when a patient refuses drug intervention (e.g., they may feel the risk of unwanted side-effects outweighs the potential benefits of taking the drug). Whilst this may feel uncomfortable to some clinicians, it does demonstrate concordant behaviour as the patient is demonstrating that they have understood the options, yet exercised their right to refuse the treatment.

Is the concordant approach more effective in terms of ensuring better use of medicines and increasing patient outcomes than other approaches? As yet, concordance has not been extensively evaluated. However, a recent systematic review of the literature related to concordance found that two-way communication between patients and professionals resulted in several benefits, including increased adherence to treatment regimens, increased health outcomes and fewer medication related problems (Cox *et al.*, 2003). Chapter 9 provides a fuller discussion of the work by Cox *et al.* and an overview of the evidence base for the concept of concordance.

To conclude, if prescribers are to realise the full potential of their role, they must base their prescribing decisions on the best available evidence. For this to happen they need to create ways to ensure they keep abreast of any new evidence relating to their area of clinical practice. By doing so they will ensure that their patients receive safe, effective treatment and also equip themselves with the knowledge, confidence and competency to fully contribute to the development and delivery of a modernising NHS.

References

Audit Commission (2001). *A Spoonful of Sugar: Medicines Management in NHS Hospitals.* London: Audit Commission.

Barber N (1995). What constitutes good prescribing? *British Medical Journal* **310**: 923–925.

Barry CA *et al.* (2000). Patients unvoiced agenda in general practice consultations: Qualitative study. *British Medical Journal* **320**: 1246–1250.

Bucher HC, Weinbacher M *et al.* (1994). Influence of method of reporting study results on decision of physicians to prescribe drugs to lower cholesterol concentration. *British Medical Journal* **309**: 761–764.

Committee on Safety of Medicines/Medicines and Healthcare products Regulatory Agency. *Monitoring the Safety and Quality of Medicines: The Yellow Card Scheme.* See http://medicines.mhra.gov.uk

Cox K *et al.* (2003). *A Systematic Review of Communication between Patients and Healthcare Professionals about Medicine-taking and Prescribing.* London: GKT Concordance Unit. King's College.

Department of Health (2000a). *Pharmacy in the Future: Implementing the NHS Plan. A Programme for Pharmacy in the National Health Service.* London: Stationery Office.

Department of Health (2000b). *Organisation with a Memory.* London: Stationery Office.

Department of Health (2000c). *The NHS Plan: A Plan for Investment, A Plan for Reform.* London: Stationery Office.

Department of Health (2003a). *Prescription Cost Analysis: England 2002.* London: Stationery Office. Available from www.doh.gov.uk/stats/pca2002.htm

Department of Health (2003b). *Prescription Cost Analysis: England 1998.* London: Stationery Office. Available from www.doh.gov.uk/stata/pca98.htm

Drummond MF *et al.* (1997). How to use an article on economic analysis of clinical practice. A: Are the results of the study valid? Users' guides to the medical literature. *Journal of the American Medical Association* **277**: 1552–1557.

Egger M *et al.* (2001). *Systematic Reviews in Healthcare: Meta-Analysis in Context.* London: *British Medical Journal* Publishing Group.

Framingham study. See www.framingham.com/heart

Gray JM (1997). *Evidence-based Healthcare.* Edinburgh: Churchill Livingstone.

Greenhalgh T (2000). *How to Read a Paper: the Basics of Evidence Based Medicine.* London: British Medical Journal books.

Jones C (2002). Research Methods (1). *The Pharmaceutical Journal* **268**: 839–841.

Jones I, Britten N (1998). Why do some patients not cash in their prescriptions? *British Journal of General Practice* **48**: 903–905.

Moore A, McQuay H (1997). *What is an NNT?* Hayward Medical Communications Ltd.

O'Brien B *et al.* (1997). How to use an article on economic analysis of clinical practice. B: What are the results and will they help me in caring for patients? Users' guides to the medical literature. *Journal of the American Medical Association* **277**: 1802–1806.

Parish PA (1973). Drug prescribing – the concern of all. *Journal of the Royal Society of Health.* Cited In: What constitutes good prescribing? (Barber N, 1995) *British Medical Journal* **310**: 923–925.

Philips C, Thompson G (1997). *What is Cost-Effectiveness?* Hayward Medical Communications Ltd.

Royal Pharmaceutical Society (1998). *From Compliance to Concordance: Achieving Shared Goals in Medicines Taking.* London: Royal Pharmaceutical Society.

Sackett DL, Rosenburg WMC *et al.* (1996). Evidence-based medicine: what it is and what it isn't. *British Medical Journal* **312**: 71–72.

Trinder L, Reynolds S (eds) (2000). *Evidence-based Practice: A Critical Appraisal.* Oxford: Blackwell Publishing.

Walley T *et al.* (ed) (2004). *Pharmacoeconomics.* Edinburgh: Churchill Livingstone.

Chapter 11

Extended/supplementary prescribing: a public health perspective

Sarah J O'Brien

In this chapter the wider, public health context of extended/supplementary prescribing is considered.

PUBLIC HEALTH

Public health is defined as 'the science and art of preventing disease, prolonging life, and promoting health through the organised efforts of society' (Acheson, 1988). Thus public health practice is focused on enhancing the health of the population as a whole, rather than necessarily treating individual patients. The definition of a population may vary with context. It might be defined geographically (e.g. a locality like a general practice population), or in terms of particular client groups (e.g. children, people on low incomes) or people with specific health needs (e.g. people with diabetes or heart disease) (Public Health/Strategic Development Directorates, 1999).

Public health personnel, working with other professional groups, undertake a variety of functions. These include monitoring the health status of the population, identifying health needs, building programmes to reduce risk and screen for early disease, controlling and preventing communicable diseases, developing policies to promote health, planning and evaluating healthcare provision, and managing and implementing change (Chief Medical Officer, 2003a).

Health inequalities are given a prominent place in the Government's public health agenda. It has been accepted for some time that there is a direct relationship between deprivation and poor health. It is a consistent finding that the less affluent in society tend to die at an earlier age than those who are wealthier (Donaldson, 2000). In a landmark publication in 1980, Sir Douglas Black and colleagues confirmed once again the existence of a gradient in mortality by social class, i.e. those in lower social classes fared worse in terms of overall mortality but also in terms of deaths from specific causes (Department of Health and Social Security (DHSS), 1980). Arguments followed about the use of social class as indices of deprivation, so that Townsend and colleagues (1987) developed a 'social index' reflecting material deprivation, from four census variables: unemployment, not owning a car, not owning a house and over-crowding. Applying this 'social index' to the population of 678 local authority wards in northern England, they found significant correlations between their index and premature deaths, chronic ill health and low birth weight. In other words, there was a measurable health gap between the people in the wealthiest wards and the people in the poorest wards. Fresh momentum has been injected into the inequalities debate with a number of publications including the report of an Independent Inquiry into Health Inequalities (Acheson, 1998), a Treasury-led Cross Cutting Review (HM Treasury and Department of Health (DoH), 2002), the National Health Services (NHS) Plan with its emphasis on tackling inequalities through more effective prevention and improved primary care for disadvantaged populations (DoH, 2002) and *Securing our Future Health: Taking a Long Term View*, which looked at NHS Spending (Wanless, 2002). Health inequalities are an intractable problem and there are no easy solutions. However, in its document *Tackling Health Inequalities – A Programme for Action* the DoH has set out plans for a 3-year programme, contributing towards the national 2010 targets to reduce the gap in infant mortality across all social groups and to raise life expectancy in the most disadvantaged areas faster than elsewhere (DoH, 2003a). A number of specific interventions will be needed amongst disadvantaged groups including a reduction in cigarette smoking, prevention and management of cardiovascular and cancer risk factors, such as poor nutrition and obesity, physical inactivity and hypertension, improving housing quality and reducing accidents both at home and on the highways. In the short-term, closing the gap on infant mortality means improving the quality of, and access to, antenatal care, reducing cigarette smoking and improving nutrition in pregnancy, preventing teenage pregnancy and supporting teenage parents, and improving housing conditions (DoH, 2003a). Obvious consequences are that delivering this ambitious national programme requires co-operation across government and that local engagement is crucial. Local solutions are needed, based on the experience and knowledge of front-line staff, and Local Strategic Partnerships will be key to delivery. Front-line workers are being given the freedom to innovate in responding to community needs through the Priorities and Planning Framework (DoH, 2003b). In a recently published consultation document from the (DoH, 2004) entitled *Standards for Better Health*, core public health standards for healthcare organisations include their responsibility to collaborate with relevant local organisations and communities to promote, protect and improve the health of the community served and narrow health inequalities (DoH, 2004).

Delivering good health for the population involves much more than simply prescribing medicines. However, where medication is needed, it is important to be familiar with the policies that guide prescribing in a public health context.

Patients and society

Prescribed medicines are the most frequently supplied treatments for NHS patients. General Practitioners (GPs) in England issue more than 660 million prescriptions every year. Additionally, there are an estimated 200 million hospital prescriptions (Smith, 2004). In considering the impact of extended/supplementary prescribing there is a balance to be struck between the benefits that it may afford for the individual patient and the effects on the population as a whole. In essence, therefore, prescribing decisions should benefit the individual without being detrimental to society as a whole. This is exemplified in the sphere of antimicrobial prescribing. Using antibiotics in one patient may influence the efficacy and efficiency of that antibiotic for use in another patient through the development of resistance.

So the needs of an individual must be balanced against the necessity to preserve the value of antimicrobial agents for the community as a whole. It should also be borne in mind that the societal impact of profligate use of antimicrobials might affect the treatment options for future generations.

Policies on antimicrobial prescribing

Antimicrobial agents are used to treat infections in individual patients and in public health interventions to control disease outbreaks (Tapsall, 2003). Policies on antimicrobial prescribing are directed towards limiting the development and further spread of antimicrobial resistance. Rationalising antimicrobial use is a complex issue, requiring commitment from clinicians and professional societies, the public, government, and international agencies (Keuleyan, 2001).

ANTIMICROBIAL RESISTANCE

The public health importance of antimicrobial resistance is the subject of much concern, debate and study. The emergence of antimicrobial resistance has, by and large, been correlated with the rise and fall of specific antimicrobial use in medical practice. However, it is generally agreed that the use of antimicrobials in veterinary clinical practice and in agriculture has also played a part. As early as 1969, the Swann Committee recommended that certain antibacterial agents should only be prescribed for veterinary use and should not be used as growth promoters (Anon, 1969).

Such is the weight attached to the public health problems posed by antimicrobial resistance that the announcement of nurse prescribing in 2001 led to a debate in the House of Lords. In particular, the Government was asked what precautions they proposed to take to guard against an increasing prevalence of antibiotic resistant organisms in the light of the Nurse Prescribing Regulations (The UK Parliament, 2002).

The term antimicrobial agent encompasses antibacterial, antifungal antiprotozoal and antiviral agents. Although the term is often used synonymously to mean 'antibiotic', in actual fact antibiotics form a subset of antimicrobial agents. Antimicrobial agents eradicate susceptible organisms but problems arise because of the resistant organisms that survive to infect other individuals. The development of antimicrobial resistance is a straightforward example of natural selection, i.e. the 'survival of the fittest' (Standing Medical Advisory Committee (SMAC) Sub-group on Antimicrobial Resistance, 1998). Resistance can arise through spontaneous, random genetic mutations, through transfer of resistance genes between organisms, or through the selection of inherently resistant species. The importance of these processes varies with organisms, antimicrobial agents and clinical situations. A description of the mechanisms of antimicrobial resistance is given in the SMACs Report *The Path of Least Resistance* (1998). Multi-resistance occurs when an organism is resistant to two or more unrelated antimicrobial agents. There is much evidence in the peer-reviewed literature of antimicrobial resistance in many organisms.

CONSEQUENCES OF ANTIMICROBIAL RESISTANCE

Most anxiety tends to be concentrated on resistance to antibacterial agents, although it should be borne in mind that similar issues are emerging with antifungal and antiviral agents. There are several consequences of antimicrobial resistance. Firstly, it may make infections more difficult to treat and treatment failures across a range of infections, and in a variety of settings, have been documented (Babin *et al.*, 2003; Bjerrum *et al.*, 2002; Davidson *et al.*, 2002; Mølbak *et al.*, 1999; Perez-Trallero *et al.*, 1990; Perez-Trallero *et al.*, 2003; Ruiz *et al.*, 2002; Vasallo *et al.*, 1998). Treatment failures, at best, necessitate the use of alternative drugs, which are often more expensive and may have unwelcome side-effects (SMAC Report, 1998). In the case of resistant tuberculosis, treatment failures can also have direct public health implications in terms of onward transmission of a resistant organism to others in the community (SMAC Report, 1998).

Secondly, the infection may be more severe. For example, there was a significant excess of deaths in Danish patients infected with antimicrobial drug-resistant *Salmonella* Typhimurium (Helms *et al.*, 2002). Similarly, it has been suggested that infection with methicillin-resistant *Staphylococcus aureus* (MRSA) is an increasing cause of mortality in England and Wales (Crowcroft, 2002; Crowcroft *et al.*, 2003). There is also evidence that infection with a resistant organism leads to a longer duration of illness (Helms *et al.*, 2002).

Another effect of antimicrobial resistance is that it may lead to increased length of hospital stay (Anon, 2002; Carmeli, 1999; Kim *et al.*, 2001; Pelletier *et al.*, 2002).

Increases in treatment and associated costs also occur in hospitals and the community (Abramson and Sexton, 1999; Carmelli *et al.*, 1999; Eandi, 1998; Kim *et al.*, 2001; Paladino *et al.*, 2002; Rubin *et al.*, 1999).

In summary, antimicrobial resistance can adversely affect patient outcome by enhancing virulence, causing a delay in administering appropriate therapy and limiting available therapy (Cosgrove, 2003).

CONTROLLING ANTIMICROBIAL RESISTANCE

If antimicrobials are viewed as a valuable public resource then a societal goal must be to minimise resistance (McGowan, 2001) and, indeed, the control of antimicrobial resistance is a major government priority. Recently, there have been two very influential expert reports, *The Path of Least Resistance* from the SMAC Sub-Group on Antimicrobial Resistance (1998) and *Resistance to antibiotics and other antimicrobial agents* from the House of Lords Select Committee on Science and Technology (1998), both of which expressed major concerns about the increasing clinical and public health importance of antimicrobial resistance. In 1999, the NHS Executive published a Health Service Circular on *Resistance to Antibiotics and Other Antimicrobial Agents* and in 2000 the DoH issued its *UK Antimicrobial Resistance Strategy and Action Plan* (2000c). A national Specialist Advisory Committee on Antimicrobial Resistance (SACAR), which has an overview of medical, veterinary and agricultural use of antimicrobials, has been created to advise the Government on future strategy.

The main aims of the Government's strategy are to reduce morbidity and mortality of infections due to antimicrobial resistant organisms and to maintain the effectiveness of antimicrobial agents in the treatment and prevention of infections in animals and man (DoH, 2000b). There are three interconnected elements – surveillance, prudent antimicrobial use and infection control. These are to be underpinned by improvements in information technology and a co-ordinated research programme.

Surveillance

Surveillance is essential in controlling antimicrobial resistance. For individual patients, and where clinical samples have been submitted for laboratory investigation, information from susceptibility testing allows informed decisions on the best therapeutic options. When the information from each individual report is collated centrally (in England by the Health Protection Agency (formerly the Public Health Laboratory Service (PHLS)), in Wales by the National Public Health Service and in Scotland by the Scottish Centre for Infection and Environmental Health) monitoring changing resistance patterns may indicate emerging problems, leading to appropriately targeted interventions and control measures. Knowledge gleaned from surveillance data concerning prevailing antimicrobial resistance patterns should also inform the development of prescribing policies (for both hospitals and the community), and thus guide empirical prescribing.

In 2002 the (then) PHLS published its first comprehensive report on antimicrobial resistance in England and Wales (PHLS, 2002). It was noted that antimicrobial susceptibility reporting was very variable: by organism, by antimicrobial agent and by NHS region. For the pathogens causing systemic infections, the most commonly reported cause of bacteraemia was *S. aureus*, of which 42% were methicillin-resistant. 55% of *Escherichia coli* organisms (the second most commonly reported cause of bacteraemia) were resistant to ampicillin/amoxicillin, 5% were resistant to ciprofloxacin and 3% were resistant to gentamicin. However, there were large regional variations in reported resistance. For enteric infections, around 20% of *Campylobacter jejuni* isolates were resistant to ciprofloxacin and two of the common *Salmonella* serotypes were prone to multiple resistance (67% of *S.* Typhimurium and 49% of *S.* Virchow). Nine percent of *Neisseria gonorrhoeae* isolates were resistant to penicillin and there were large regional variations in penicillin, tetracycline and ciprofloxacin resistance. Up-to-date information on important publications can be found on the Health Protection Agency's website at: http://www.hpa.org.uk/infections/topics_az/antimicrobial_resistance/menu.htm

The data presented in the PHLS report (2002) illustrate the value of antimicrobial susceptibility testing in informing antimicrobial prescribing. Susceptibility patterns for many pathogens, especially respiratory tract pathogens, may change over short distances making local medical microbiology services essential for rational prescribing decisions (SMAC Report, 1998). Medical microbiologists can advise on appropriate specimen collection and there are often local protocols providing guidance on the types of specimens that need to be obtained in particular clinical situations, including the timing in relation to transport to the laboratory. Knowledge of local resistance patterns gained through diagnostic testing then helps to guide local antimicrobial prescribing policies. It is incumbent on prescribers to familiarise themselves with local antimicrobial resistance patterns and local antimicrobial prescribing policies. All Trusts and Primary Care Trusts (PCTs) are required to implement and review local policies and guidelines on appropriate antimicrobial use on an annual basis. In the SMAC Report (1998) it was noted that guidelines should be evidence-based, including the strength of that evidence, and bear the date on which they were developed. They should contain information on the agent, dosage, frequency and length of course. Finally, they should indicate where local policy varied from national advice.

As well as understanding what is happening to micro-organisms with respect to antimicrobial resistance, there is also a need to gather better data on antimicrobial usage in the UK and to better correlate information on antimicrobial usage patterns, trends in antimicrobial resistance and clinical disease in both the human and animal populations due to antimicrobial resistant organisms. Collation of prescribing and clinical data will take place as part of the new NHS Health Information Strategy and the Department for Environment, Food and Rural Affairs is leading on resistance issues as they relate to the animal population. Tighter controls on the use of antimicrobials in both medical and veterinary clinical practice are welcome and are already underway in the UK. However, agricultural and clinical practice (both veterinary and medical) elsewhere in the world will continue to have an impact on resistant bacteria identified in the UK through foreign travel and global trade.

Controlling healthcare-associated infections as well as antimicrobial resistance, is now a priority (Chief Medical Officer, 2003b) and compulsory surveillance systems for *S. aureus* bacteraemias, including MRSA, in England was established in 2001 (DoH, 2001; Duckworth *et al.*, 2002), and there are plans to include certain other antimicrobial resistant infections (DoH, 2003c).

Prudent antimicrobial prescribing

The clinical prescribing sub-group of the Interdepartmental Steering Group on Resistance to Antibiotics and other Antimicrobial Agents in its report on *Optimising the clinical use of antimicrobials: report and recommendations for further work* (2001), defined prudent antimicrobial prescribing as:

> The use of antimicrobials in the most appropriate way for the treatment or prevention of human infectious diseases, having regard to the diagnosis (or presumed diagnosis), evidence of clinical effectiveness, likely benefits, safety, cost (in comparison with alternative choices), and propensity for the emergence of resistance. The most appropriate way implies that the choice, route, dose, frequency and duration of administration have been rigorously determined

They considered that prudent meant both 'less' (they deemed that there was still scope to reduce unnecessary use of antimicrobials) and 'appropriate' (i.e. the right dose of the right antibiotic, administered via the most appropriate route for the right length of time to produce a clinical cure, whilst minimising side-effects and the development of resistance).

A number of ways to optimise antimicrobial prescribing in clinical practice has been developed. In its report *The Path of Least Resistance* SMAC (1998) published 'four things you can do'. These were:

- '*No prescribing of antibiotics for simple coughs and colds*
- *No prescribing of antibiotics for viral sore throats*
- *Limit prescribing for uncomplicated cystitis to 3 days in otherwise fit women*
- *Limit prescribing of antibiotics over the telephone to exceptional cases*'

The majority (around 80%) of antimicrobial prescribing takes place in primary care and approximately half of these prescriptions have been issued for respiratory tract infections. Yet the evidence that there are benefits from prescribing anti-biotics for sore throats (Ben-David, 2002; Hirschmann, 2002), sinusitis (Leggett, 2004) and acute otitis media (Darrow et al., 2003; Schilder et al., 2004) is fairly small. In certain circumstances, empirical therapy for a range of infections from acute bacterial rhinosinusitis to cystitis may be justified, but this also illustrates the importance of carefully evaluating symptoms and employing appropriate diagnos-tic tests (Contopoulos-Ioannidis et al., 2003; Garau, 2003; Leibovitz, 2003; Nicolle, 2003). A useful resource for guiding diagnosis and management is the 'Prodigy' guidelines, a computerised decision support system, available on the worldwide web at www.prodigy.nhs.uk. 'Clinical Evidence' comprises a compilation of the best available evidence for healthcare and is a key part of the National electronic Library for Health, available at www.nelh.nhs.uk/clinicalevidence. It summarises the current state of knowledge on, and reservations about, the prevention and treatment of clinical conditions, based on comprehensive searches and appraisal of the scientific literature. It does not provide clinical guidelines but useful synthe-ses on state-of-the-art knowledge about various common clinical conditions are helpful background information. Management of infection guidelines for primary care, which can be adopted for local use, have been developed by the Health Protection Agency and are available at http://www.hpa.org.uk/infections/topics_az/antimicro-bial_resistance/guidance.htm.

Another important consideration for the prescriber is to appreciate when a patient may benefit from a medical opinion. This is analogous to the situation when a GP may seek the help of a specialist hospital colleague.

Kumar and colleagues (2003) recently published a study concerning GPs' anti-biotic prescribing habits for sore throat. They found that the GPs they surveyed were unsure which patients were likely to benefit from antibiotics. They tended to prescribe for patients who they judged to be more unwell and for those from more deprived backgrounds because of fears about complications. They were also more likely to prescribe in pressurised clinical situations. However, the encouraging news is that antimicrobial prescribing policies do seem to work to change clini-cians' behaviour (Feucht, 2003; McNulty, 2001; Tiley et al., 2003). It has been sug-gested that multidisciplinary approaches including participation from physicians, nurses, pharmacists and infection control staff are successful (Gross, 2001; Pflomm, 2002). However, whilst alterations in prescribing behaviour have been observed, the evidence that this has yet had an effect on antimicrobial resistance is more limited (Wilton et al., 2002).

In addition to ensuring that professionals are enabled to prescribe antimicrobials optimally in clinical practice, the Government's strategy also includes provision of better diagnostic and antimicrobial susceptibility testing methods, providing more rapid information to prescribers, whilst safeguarding surveillance data.

Another key component of the strategy is managing public expectations. This recognises that patients, too, have a role in reducing antimicrobial resistance by not expecting inappropriate treatment (Holmes et al., 2003). Macfarlane and col-leagues (1997a) provided a graphic illustration of this. They surveyed 1014 patients who had recently consulted their GP with an acute lower respiratory tract infection. Of the 787 patients who replied to the questionnaire, 656 of the 662 patients who attributed their symptoms to an infection thought that antibiotics would help. Moreover, 564 patients wanted an antibiotic, 561 expected to receive one and 146 actually requested one. In the SMAC Report (1998), attention was drawn to the need for a public campaign to handle patients' expectations and to influence their attitudes towards antimicrobial agents. The Government has backed the recommendation with a national public information campaign (DoH, 2002a; DoH, 2002b; DoH, 2002c). Evidence shows that where patients are involved in decision-making about their care, coupled with better information about their condition, and the advantages and disadvantages of antimicrobial therapy, access to and completion of appropriate antimicrobial therapy is improved (Davey et al., 2002). Re-consultation rates may also go down (Macfarlane et al., 1997).

Infection control

This part of the Government's strategy is aimed at reducing the spread of infection in general (and hence limiting the need for using antimicrobial agents) and of antimicrobial resistant organisms in particular. In the US it has been estimated that around 30–40% of resistant infections occur through cross-infection, 20–25% through selective antimicrobial pressure, 20–25% through the introduction of new pathogens, the remainder being unknown (McGowan, 2001). In a large hospital survey in the UK, it was estimated that around 8% of in-patients presented with one or more hospital-acquired infections during the in-patient period (Plowman et al., 2001). The estimated costs of these infections to the hospital sector were in the region of £930 million.

Despite the importance of healthcare-associated infection, it does not seem to have been afforded the priority by the NHS that it deserves. A plethora of guidance and guideline documents and health service circulars has been issued on the subject over the last few years. In his report *Winning Ways – Working together to reduce healthcare-associated infection in England* the Chief Medical Officer (2003b) has re-affirmed commitment to tackling this intractable problem. He outlines the need for senior management commitment; local infrastructure and systems, making it clear that dealing with healthcare-associated infection must not be left to clinical staff alone. Each organisation providing NHS services is to have a Director of Infection Prevention and Control who will, amongst other things, oversee and implement local infection control policies, be responsible for the Infection Control Team and report directly to the Chief Executive and the Board. Importantly, they will have the authority to challenge inappropriate clinical hygiene, as well as antimicrobial prescribing decisions, and they will be an integral member of the organisation's clinical governance and patient safety groups. A public annual report must also be produced. One of the seven action areas in the Chief Medical Officer's report relates to high standards of hygiene in clinical practice. Detailed guidelines for preventing hospital-acquired infection have been published (Pratt et al., 2001) and are also available at the *epic* (evidence-based practice in infection control) website http://www.epic.tvu.ac.uk. Prudent antimicrobial prescribing in hospitals is also referred to in *Winning Ways – Working together to reduce healthcare-associated infection in England* (Chief Medical Officer, 2003b), with the development of the hospital pharmacy initiative (DoH, 2003d) and illustrates how closely intertwined are the dual themes of prudent prescribing and infection control.

The Government is concerned to strengthen infection control practices not only in hospitals but also in the community. This is in recognition of the fact that there are more beds in the community, with patients staying in them for longer, than in hospital, coupled with increasing numbers of nursing and residential homes and hospices. The volume and types of surgical procedures being carried out in primary care are increasing and the shorter hospital stays enabled by minimally invasive surgery mean that infections previously detected and dealt with in hospital are now being identified and managed in the community (Communicable Disease Surveillance Centre, 2002). The National Institute for Clinical Excellence (NICE) (2003) published detailed guidelines on preventing healthcare-associated infection in primary and community care in 2003. These were developed by Thames Valley University under the sponsorship of the National Collaborating Centre for Nursing and Supportive Care (Pellowe *et al.*, 2003) and are also available on the *epic* website at http://www.epic.tvu.ac.uk.

Developmental standards proposed by the Government in its document *Standards for Better Health* (DoH, 2004) include that healthcare be provided in well-designed environments that are appropriate for safe and effective delivery of treatment, care or specific functions, including effective control of healthcare-associated infections. The Commission for Healthcare Audit and Inspection will be responsible for developing detailed criteria underpinning these standards and for inspecting NHS delivery and performance against all core and developmental standards. This high profile approach is indicative of the priority afforded to infection control.

Notifiable and other communicable diseases

Under the Public Health (Control of Disease Act) 1984 and the Public Health (Infectious Diseases) Regulations 1988 certain infectious diseases are notifiable by law. Under current legislation the legal duty to notify rests with a doctor. If follows, therefore, that medical colleagues need to be informed of any diseases required to be notified to the Proper Officer of the local authority, which is usually a Consultant in Communicable Disease Control in the local health protection unit. Notification forms are available from the local authority and a fee is payable for each notification. The Public Health (Control of Disease) Act 1984 requires that the following information is disclosed: patient's name, age, sex and address. The legal duty to notify these personal details has not been superseded by the Data Protection Act (McTigue, 2003). Notification should take place on clinical suspicion that a patient is suffering from a notifiable disease. It need not await laboratory confirmation. Indeed, the delays inherent in obtaining a laboratory diagnosis might mean that secondary spread has already occurred.

The list of notifiable diseases, which can be found in the British National Formulary (BNF), includes food poisoning. In 1992, the Advisory Committee on the Microbiological Safety of Food defined food poisoning as any condition of an infectious or toxic nature, caused by, or thought to be caused by contaminated food or water (ACMSF, 1992). Although treatment, other than supportive measures, is not usually recommended for patients with uncomplicated gastroenteritis, symptoms may herald an outbreak of food poisoning. Useful advice on when to contact the local consultant in communicable disease control is contained in the Communicable Disease Control Handbook (Hawker *et al.*, 2001).

The purpose of notification is to allow the Proper Officer to take prompt public health action and institute control measures as soon as possible, within the incubation period of the disease in question, in order to prevent more people from becoming unwell. These control measures may include vaccination.

Vaccination policy

The childhood vaccination programme represents one of the most successful public health interventions of modern times. Diseases like poliomyelitis and diphtheria, which were still major child killers as late as the 1950s, are now virtually eliminated. In May 1980, less than 200 years after Edward Jenner demonstrated that vaccination with material from cowpox protected against the development of smallpox, the World Health Assembly accepted that smallpox had been eradicated from the world (DoH, 1996). Now, ironically, concerns arise from its potential use as a bioterrorist agent.

The aims of vaccination programmes are to achieve herd immunity in the susceptible population against those diseases which are spread from person-to-person, e.g. measles, and to protect everyone against infections from other sources, e.g. tetanus (Hawker *et al.*, 2001). These aims are met either through inducing active immunity, through the use of inactivated or live, attenuated organisms or their products, or through inducing passive immunity by means of immunoglobulins. Active immunity is long-lasting, whereas passive immunity, although offering immediate protection, is short-lived. Some of the considerations in offering vaccinations are outlined below, but detailed guidance is available on the DoH website at http://www.dh.gov.uk/PublicationsAndStatistics/Publications/PublicationsPolicy AndGuidance/PublicationsPolicyAndGuidanceArticle/fs/en?CONTENT_ID= 4072977&chk=87uz6M> where updated chapters from the *Green Book* on Immunisation against Infectious Disease (DoH *et al.*, 1996) are posted from time to time. The replacement chapters represent current DoH recommendations and should be followed in place of the 1996 version. Communications from the Chief Medical Officer or the Chief Nursing Officer regarding vaccination should be kept on file for future reference.

CONSENT FOR VACCINATION

Consent must always be obtained before vaccinating a child and parents must always feel that they have been fully included in the decision. Consent is needed at the time of each immunisation, after the child has been judged to be a suitable candidate including being fit enough to receive the vaccine (DoH *et al.*, 1996). Consent that has been obtained before the child was brought in to receive the vaccine is an agreement for the child to be included in the programme. Consent should still be sought for the vaccination to be given, and written consent provides a permanent record.

VACCINES: STORAGE, DISTRIBUTION AND DISPOSAL

Detailed instructions can be found in Chapter 4 of the *Green Book*. In essence, vaccines should be stored according to the Manufacturer's instructions. They should be kept on the shelves in a designated vaccine refrigerator, the temperature of which can be constantly monitored. Careful attention should be paid to the shelf-life, so that vaccines that have reached their expiry date should not be used, and written procedures for storage, distributions and disposal of vaccines should be audited regularly.

VACCINES: INDICATIONS AND CONTRAINDICATIONS

There are some conditions that increase the risk of complications from an infectious disease, and people with these conditions should be immunised as a priority (DoH *et al.*, 1996). These conditions include asthma, chronic lung disease, congenital heart disease, Down's syndrome, small for dates babies, babies born prematurely and people with human immunodeficiency virus (HIV) infection. People with no spleen, or who have functional hyposplenism, are at increased risk from certain bacterial infections, like *Streptococcus pneumoniae*, and should receive appropriate cover. Haemodialysis patients are at increased risk of hepatitis B and hepatitis C, and, following vaccination, their hepatitis B markers should be monitored regularly and re-immunisation offered as needed.

General contraindications to vaccination include an acute febrile illness, and a definite history of a severe local or general reaction to a preceding dose of a vaccine. Where there is doubt about what might constitute a severe local or general reaction advice can be sought from clinical colleagues like a Consultant Paediatrician, Consultant in Communicable Disease Control or the District Immunisation Co-ordinator. Definitions of severe local and general reactions to vaccination are given in Chapter 7 of the *Green Book*.

It is not advisable to give live virus vaccines to pregnant women because of the theoretical possibility of harming the fetus. However, where there is a significant risk that a pregnant woman has been exposed to a disease like poliomyelitis or yellow fever, the indications for vaccination outweigh the potential risk to the fetus. Administration of live virus vaccines is also contraindicated in certain groups of patients with impaired immunity, e.g. those undergoing treatment for malignancy, recent bone marrow transplant recipients, those on high dose steroids or other immunosuppressants, and people with impaired cell-mediated immunity like those with HIV infection. There are specific contraindications to individual vaccines and all those prepared to administer vaccines should ensure that they have read the most up-to-date information from the manufacturer, and have studied the relevant chapters in the *Green Book*, checking for updates on the DoH website.

VACCINATION PROCEDURES

Covered in depth in Chapter 5 of the *Green Book*, a major consideration is that, before administering any vaccine, the individual should have received training and be proficient in the appropriate techniques including, subcutaneous, intramuscular and intradermal injection techniques. The individual must have made appropriate arrangements for dealing with anaphylactic (see Chapter 10 of the *Green Book*) and other immediate reactions. The person administering the vaccine should have familiarised themselves with the procedures when they need to give more than one vaccine at the same time. Those performing vaccination should also know about and understand the procedures for reporting adverse reactions through the *Yellow Card* scheme to the Medicines Control Agency.

THE CHILDHOOD VACCINATION PROGRAMME

The current immunisation schedule is as follows (Hawker *et al.*, 2001):

- *For neonates*: Bacille Calmette-Guérin (BCG) and Hepatitis B vaccinations may be indicated for certain groups

- *For children at 2, 3 and 4 months of age*: three doses of primary course of diphtheria/tetanus/pertussis (DTP), oral polio, *Haemophilus influenzae* b (Hib), Meningococcus C

- *For children at 12 to 15 months of age*: one dose primary course of measles/mumps/rubella (MMR I)

- *For children aged 3 to 5 years*: one booster dose of diphtheria/tetanus (low dose) (DT), oral polio, measles/mumps/rubella (MMR II)

- *For children aged 10 to 14 years*: BCG

- *For children aged 13 to 18 years*: booster doses of tetanus/diphtheria (low dose) (Td), oral polio

- *For adults*: booster doses of tetanus and polio, if appropriate, and vaccines for lifestyle/occupational risks

- *For adults over 65 years*: influenza.

Influenza and pneumococcus vaccines may be recommended at any age for special medical risk groups, and vaccines offering protection for overseas travel may also be indicated at any age (although some have a lower age limit).

The UK immunisation schedule changes from time to time, on advice from an independent expert advisory committee, the Joint Committee on Vaccination and Immunisation.

PROTECTING THE HEALTH OF TRAVELLERS OVERSEAS

In 2001 the DoH published the second edition of the sister companion to the *Green Book* (DoH *et al.*, 2001). *Health Information for Overseas Travel* or the *Yellow Book* as it has become known is a concise and authoritative source of information about the common health risks faced by overseas travellers and the ways to reduce them. Like the *Green Book* it is also available through the DoH website at http://www.archive.official-documents.co.uk/document/doh/hinfo/travel02.htm.

Final thoughts

Although much of this chapter has focused on antimicrobial resistance and vaccination, the principles outlined with regard to prudent prescribing apply equally well to drugs other than antimicrobials. *Building on the Best* (DoH, 2003e) extends patient choice through a number of measures, including easier availability of repeat prescriptions and extending the range of over the counter medicines that will be available for purchase without a prescription. Thus prescribers also need to be alert to the fact that patients might have obtained other medicines over the counter and that these might interact with prescribed medication. And in McTigue's (2004) useful summary on managing clinical risks she provides some practical suggestions for managing the risks associated with repeat prescribing. Implementing extended/supplementary prescribing is intended to benefit individual patients and society as a whole.

References

Abramson MA, Sexton DJ (1999). Nosocomial methicillin-resistant and methicillin-susceptible *Staphylococcus aureus* primary bacteremia: at what costs? *Infection Control and Hospital Epidemiology* **20**: 408–411.

Acheson D (1988). Public Health in England: *Report of the Committee of Inquiry into the Future Development of the Public Health Function.* Department of Health.

Acheson D (1998). *Report of the Independent Inquiry into Inequalities in Health.* (Chairman: Sir Donald Acheson). London: The Stationery Office.

Advisory Committee on the Microbiological Safety of Food (1992).

Anon (1969). *Report of the Joint Committee on the Use of Antimicrobials in Animal Husbandry and Veterinary Medicine (Swann Committee).* London: HMSO.

Anon (2002). The cost of antibiotic resistance: effect of resistance among *Staphylococcus aureus, Klebsiella pneumoniae, Acinetobacter baumannii,* and *Pseudmonas aeruginosa* on length of hospital stay. *Infection Control and Hospital Epidemiology* **23**: 106–108.

Babin E, Lemarchand V, Moreau S, Goullet de Rugy M, Valdazo A, Bequignon A (2003). Failure of antibiotic therapy in acute otitis media. *Journal of Laryngology and Otology* **117**: 173–176.

Ben-David D, Rubinstein E (2002). Appropriate use of antibiotics for respiratory infections: review of recent statements and position papers. *Current Opinion in Infectious Diseases* **15**: 151–156.

Bjerrum L, Dessau RB, Hallas J (2002). Treatment failures after antibiotic therapy of uncomplicated urinary tract infections. A prescription database study. *Scandinavian Journal of Primary Healthcare* **20**: 97–101.

Carmeli Y, Troillet N, Karchmer AW, Samore MH (1999). Health and economic outcomes of antibiotic resistance in *Pseudomonas aeruginosa. Archives of Internal Medicine* **159**: 1127–1132.

Chief Medical Officer (2003a). *Public health in England: What is Public Health?* (on-line) Available at http://www.doh.gov.uk/cmo/publichealth/whatis.htm (accessed 31 January 2004).

Chief Medical Officer (2003b). *Winning Ways – Working together to Reduce Healthcare Associated Infection in England.* A report from the Chief Medical Officer. London: Department of Health.

Communicable Disease Surveillance Centre (2002). *Infection Control in the Community Study.* Public Health Laboratory Service.

Contopoulos-Ioannidis DG, Ioannidis JP, Lau J (2003). Acute sinusitis in children: current treatment strategies. *Paediatric Drugs* **5**: 71–80.

Cosgrove SE, Carmeli Y (2003). The impact of antimicrobial resistance on health and economic outcomes. *Clinical Infectious Diseases* **36**: 1433–1437.

Crowcroft NS, Catchpole M (2002). Mortality from methicillin resistant *Staphylococcus aureus* in England and Wales: analysis of death certificates. *British Medical Journal* **325**: 1390–1391.

Crowcroft NS, Lamagni TL, Rooney C, Catchpole M, Duckworth G (2003). Mortality from methicillin resistant *Staphylococcus aureus* (electronic response to Howard *et al*. Mortality from methicillin resistant *Staphylococcus aureus*). *British Medical Journal*. http://www.bmj.com/cgi/eletters/326/7387/501/a#30165 (accessed 5 February 2004).

Davidson R, Cavalcanti R, Brunton JL, Bast DJ, de Azavedo JC, Kibsey *et al.* (2002). Resistance to levofloxacin and failure of treatment of pneumococcal pneumonia. *New England Journal of Medicine* **346**: 747–750.

Darrow DH, Dash N, Derkay CS (2003). Otitis media: concepts and controversies. *Current Opinion in Otolaryngology & Head and Neck Surgery* **11**: 416–423.

Davey P, Pagliari C, Hayes A (2002). The patient's role in the spread and control of bacterial resistance to antibiotics. *Clinical Microbiology and Infection* **8(suppl 2)**: 43–68.

Department of Health, Welsh Office, Scottish Office Department of Health, DHSS (Northern Ireland) (1996). *Immunisation against Infectious Disease – Edward Jenner Bicentenary Edition*. (Salibury, DM and Begg, NT). London: HMSO (also known as the 'Green Book').

Department of Health, National Assembly for Wales, Scottish Executive Health Department, DHSS PS (Northern Ireland), Public Health Laboratory Service Communicable Disease Surveillance Centre (2001). *Health Information for Overseas Travel*. London: The Stationery Office (also known as the 'Yellow Book').

Department of Health (2000a). *The NHS Plan – A Plan for Investment. A Plan for Reform. A Summary (Cm4818-I)*. London: Department of Health.

Department of Health (2000b). *UK Antimicrobial Resistance Strategy and Action Plan*. London: Department of Health.

Department of Health (2001). *Surveillance of Healthcare Associated Infections*. *CMO's Update* **30**: 6.

Department of Health (2002a). *Public Education Campaign on Antimicrobial Resistance – Letter from the Communicable Diseases Branch on Phase 2 of the Antimicrobial Resistance Campaign*. Available at http://www.dh.gov.uk/ Policy And Guidance/HealthAndSocialCareTopics/AntimicrobialResistance / Antimicrobial ResistanceGeneralInformation/AntimicrobialResistanceGeneralArticle/fs/en?CO NTENT_ID=4002076&chk=dQckXR (accessed 18 February 2004).

Department of Health (2002b). *Antibiotics – Don't Wear Me Out*. Available at http://www.dh.gov.uk/assetRoot/04/01/88/73/04018873.pdf (accessed 18 February 2004).

Department of Health (2002c). *Antibiotics Don't Work on Colds or Most Coughs and Sore Throats*. Available at http://www.dh.gov.uk/assetRoot/04/01/88/74/04018874.pdf (accessed 18 February 2004).

Department of Health (2003a). *Tackling Health Inequalities – A Programme for Action*. London: Department of Health.

Department of Health (2003b). *Improvement, Expansion and Reform – The Next 3 Years: Priorities and Planning Framework 2003–2006*. Available at http://www.dh.gov.uk/assetRoot/04/07/02/02/04070202.pdf (accessed 22 February 2004).

Department of Health (2003c). *Surveillance of Healthcare Associated Infections*. London: Department of Health. (Professional Letter. Chief Medical Officer: PLCMO (2003) 4); (Professional Letter. Chief Nursing Officer: PLCNO (2003) 4.) Available at http://www.dh.gov.uk/assetRoot/04/01/34/10/04013410.pdf (accessed 20 February 2004).

Department of Health (2003d). *Hospital Pharmacy Initiative for Promoting Prudent Use of Antibiotics in Hospitals*. London: Department of Health (Professional Letter. Chief Medical Officer: PLCMO (2003) 3.) Available at http://www.doh.gov.uk/cmo/letters.htm (accessed 2 February 2004).

Department of Health (2003e). *Building on the Best – Choice, Responsiveness and Equity in the NHS. A Summary*. London: Department of Health.

Department of Health (2004). *Standards for Better Health – Healthcare Standards for Services under the NHS. A Consultation*. London: Department of Health.

Department of Health and Social Security (1980). *Inequalities in Health: Report of a Research Working Group (the Black Report)*. London: HMSO.

Donaldson LJ, Donaldson RJ (2000). *Essential Public Health* 2nd edn. Newbury: Petroc Press (LibraPharm Ltd.), pp. 131–134.

Duckworth G, Cookson B, Pearson A, Crowcroft N (2002). Surveillance for *S. aureus* bacteraemias is compulsory. *British Medical Journal* **324**: 240–241.

Eandi M, Zara GP (1998). Economic impact of resistance in the community. *International Journal of Clinical Practice* **95(suppl)**: 27–38.

Feucht CL, Rice LB (2003). An interventional program to improve antibiotic use. *Annals of Pharmacotherapy* **37**: 646–651.

Garau J, Dagan R (2003). Accurate diagnosis and appropriate treatment of acute bacterial rhinosinusitis: minimizing bacterial resistance. *Clinical Therapeutics* **25**: 1936–1951.

Gross PA, Pujat D (2001). Implementing practice guidelines for appropriate antimicrobial usage: a systematic review. *Medical Care* **39(suppl 2)**: II55–II69.

Hawker J, Begg N, Blair I, Reintjes R, Weinberg J (2001). *Communicable Disease Control Handbook* 1st edn. Oxford: Blackwell Science, pp. 248–249.

Helms M, Vastrup P, Gerner-Smidt P, Mølbak K (2002). Excess mortality associated with antimicrobial drug-resistant *Salmonella* typhimurium. *Emerging Infectious Diseases* **8**: 490–495.

HM Treasury, Department of Health (2002). *Tackling Health Inequalities – Summary of the 2002 Cross-Cutting Review*. London: Department of Health.

Hirschmann JV (2002). Antibiotics for common respiratory tract infections in adults. *Archives of Internal Medicine* **162**: 256–264.

Holmes JH, Metlay J, Holmes WC, Mikanatha N (2003). Developing a patient intervention to reduce antibiotic overuse. *Proceedings of AMIA Symposium*, 864.

House of Lords Select Committee on Science and Technology (1998). *Resistance to Antibiotics and Other Antimicrobial Agents*. 7th Report 1997–1998, HL Paper 81, 17–3–1998.

Keuleyan E, Gould M (2001). Key issues in developing antibiotic policies: from an institutional level to Europe-wide. European Study Group on Antibiotic Policy (ESGAP), Subgroup III. *Clinical Microbiology and Infection* **7(suppl 6)**: 16–21.

Kim T, Oh PI, Simor AE (2001). The economic impact of methicillin-resistant *Staphylococcus aureus* in Canadian hospitals. *Infection Control and Hospital Epidemiology* **22**: 99–104.

Kumar S, Little P, Britten N (2003). Why do General Practitioners prescribe antibiotics for sore throat? Grounded theory interview study. *British Medical Journal* **326**: 138.

Leggett JE (2004). Acute sinusitis. When-and when not-to prescribe antibiotics. *Postgraduate Medicine* **115**: 13–19.

Liebovitz E (2003). Acute otitis media in pediatric medicine: current issues in epidemiology, diagnosis and management. *Paediatric Drugs* **5(suppl 1)**: 1–12.

Macfarlane J, Holmes W, Macfarlane R, Britten N (1997a). Influence of patients' expectations on antibiotic management of acute lower respiratory tract illness in general practice: questionnaire study. *British Medical Journal* **315**: 1211–1214.

Macfarlane JT, Holmes WF *et al.* (1997b). Reducing reconsultations for acute lower respiratory tract illness with an information leaflet: a randomised controlled study of patients in primary care. *British Journal of General Practice* **47**: 719–722.

McGowan JE Jr. (2001). Economic impact of antimicrobial resistance. *Emerging Infectious Diseases* **7**: 286–292.

McNulty CA (2001). Optimising antibiotic prescribing in primary care. *International Journal of Antimicrobial Agents* **18**: 329–333.

McTigue A, Williams S (2003). *Have Confidence in Confidence Alone*. MPS Casebook **11(4)**: 8–10. Available at http://www.mps.org.uk (accessed 22 February 2004).

McTigue A (2004). *Taking Stock: Risk and Remedy*. MPS Casebook **12(1)**: 8–10. Available at http://www.mps.org.uk (accessed 22 February 2004).

Mølbak K, Baggesen DL, Aarestrup FM *et al.* (1999). An outbreak of multidrug-resistant, quinolone-resistant *Salmonella enterica* serotype Typhimurium DT104. *New England Journal of Medicine* **341**: 1420–1425.

National Institute for Clinical Excellence (2003). Infection Control: prevention of healthcare-associated infection in primary and community care. Available at http://www.nice.org.uk/pdf/CG2fullguidelineinfectioncontrol.pdf (accessed 20 February 2004).

NHS Executive (1999). *Resistance to Antibiotics and Other Antimicrobial Agents. Health Service Circular 1999/049*. London: Department of Health, 5–3–1999.

Nicolle LE (2003). Empirical treatment of acute cystitis in women. *International Journal of Antimicrobial Agents* **22**: 1–6.

Niemann J, Mølbak K, Engberg J, Aarrestrup FM, Wegener HC (2001). Longer duration of illness among *Campylobacter* patients treated with fluoroquinolones. In: Abstracts of the 11th International Workshop on *Campylobacter*, Helicobacter and related Organisms. September 1–5, 2001. Freiburg, Germany. *International Journal of Medical Microbiology* **291(suppl 31)**: 108.

Paladino JA, Sunderlin JL, Price CS, Schentag JJ (2002). Economic consequences of antimicrobial resistance. *Surgical Infections (Larchmt)* **3**: 259–267.

Pelletier SJ, Raymond DP, Crabtree TD, Gleason TG, Pruett TL, Sawyer RG (2002). Outcome analysis of intra-abdominal infection with resistant gram-positive organisms. *Surgical Infections* **3**: 11–19.

Pellowe CM, Pratt RJ, Harper P, Loveday HP, Robinson N, Jones SR *et al.* (2003). Evidence-based guidelines for preventing healthcare-associated infections in primary and community care in England. *Journal of Hospital Infection* **55(suppl 2)**: S2–S127.

Perez-Trallero E, Garcia-Arenzana JM, Jimenez JA, Peris A (1990). Therapeutic failure and selection of resistance to quinolones in a case of pneumococcal pneumonia treated with ciprofloxacin. *European Journal of Clinical Microbiology and Infectious Diseases* **9**: 905–906.

Perez-Trallero E, Marimon JM, Iglesias L, Larruskain J (2003). Fluoroquinolone and macrolide treatment failure in pneumococcal pneumonia and selection of multidrug-resistant isolates. *Emerging Infectious Diseases* **9**: 1159–1162.

Pflomm JM (2002). Strategies for minimizing antimicrobial resistance. *American Journal of Health-System Pharmacy* **59(suppl 3)**: S12–S15.

PHLS (2002). *Antimicrobial Resistance in 2000: England and Wales*. London: Public Health Laboratory Service.

Plowman R, Graves N, Griffin MA, Roberts JA, Swan AV, Cookson B *et al.* (2001). The rate and cost of hospital-acquired infections occurring in patients admitted to selected specialties of a district general hospital in England and the national burden imposed. *Journal of Hospital Infection* **47**: 198–209.

Pratt RJ, Pellowe C, Loveday HP, Robinson N, Smith GW, Barrett S *et al.* (2001). The epic project: developing national evidence-based guidelines for preventing healthcare associated infections. Phase I: Guidelines for preventing hospital-acquired infections. Department of Health (England). *Journal of Hospital Infection* **47(suppl)**: S3–S82.

Public Health/Strategic Development Directorates (1999). Public Health Practice Resource Pack. NHS Executive.

Rubin RJ, Harrington CA, Poon A, Dietrich K, Greene JA, Moiduddin A (1999). The economic impact of *Staphylococcus aureus* infection in New York City hospitals. *Emerging Infectious Diseases* **5**: 9–17.

Ruiz ME, Guerrero IC, Tuazon CU (2002). Endocarditis caused by methicillin-resistant *Staphylococcus aureus*: treatment failure with linezolid. *Clinical Infectious Diseases* **35**: 1018–1020.

Schilder AG, Lok W, Rovers MM (2004). International perspectives on management of acute otitis media: a qualitative review. *International Journal of Pediatric Otorhinolaryngology* **68**: 29–36.

Smith J (2004). *Building a safer NHS for patients – Improving Medication Safety: A Report by the Chief Pharmaceutical Officer*. Department of Health (on-line). Available at http://www.doh.gov.uk/buildsafenhs/medicationsafety/medication-safety.pdf (accessed 03 February 2004).

Standing Medical Advisory Committee Sub-group on Antimicrobial Resistance (1998). *The Path of Least Resistance*. London: Department of Health.

Tapsall JW (2003). Monitoring antimicrobial resistance for public health action. *Communicable Diseases Intelligence* **27(suppl)**: S70–S74.

The Interdepartmental Steering Group on Resistance to Antibiotics and other Antimicrobial Agents – Clinical Prescribing Subgroup (2001). *Optimising the Clinical Use of Antimicrobials: Report and Recommendations for Further Work*. Department of Health (on-line). Available at http://www.doh.gov.uk/sacar/pdfs/clinicalprescribingrpt.pdf (accessed 5 February 2004).

The United Kingdom Parliament (2002). Lords Hansard text for 24 Jan 2002 (220124–21) (on-line). Available at http://www.publications.parliament.uk/pa/ld200102/ldhansrd/vo020124/text/20124-21.htm (accessed 04 February 2004).

Tiley SM, MacDonald JJ, Doherty PL, Ferguson JK, Fergusson JE (2003). Active promotion of antibiotic guidelines: an intensive program. *Communicable Diseases Intelligence* **27(suppl)**: S13–S18.

Townsend P, Phillimore P, Beattie A (1987). *Deprivation and Health: Inequality and the North*. Beckenham: Croom Helm.

Vasallo FJ, Martin-Rabadan IP, Alcala L *et al.* (1998). Failure of ciprofloxacin therapy for invasive nontyphoidal salmonellosis. *Clinical Infectious Diseases* **26**: 535–536.

Wanless D (2002). *Securing our Future Health: Taking a Long Term View*. London: HM Treasury.

Wilton P, Smith R, Coast J, Millar M (2002). Strategies to contain the emergence of antimicrobial resistance: a systematic review of effectiveness and cost-effectiveness. *Journal of Health Services Research & Policy* **7**: 111–117.

Chapter 12

Calculation skills

Alison G Eggleton

INTRODUCTION

In the publications, Maintaining Competence in Prescribing (National Prescribing Centre (NPC), 2001; 2003) the NPC has developed competence frameworks for nurse and pharmacist prescribers. Both documents contain a section on prescribing safely in which one of the elements is 'check doses and calculations to ensure accuracy and safety'. Anyone who is to check calculations performed by others must first be competent to perform such calculations. This is the most obvious element of the framework calling for competence in calculation skills. However, there are other skills called for in which competence in calculations is implicit in performing the role of a prescriber. For example, the prescriber will have access to a drug budget and must make sure that their prescribing is cost-effective. The prescriber should understand the pharmacokinetics of medicines and how changes such as age and renal impairment affect dosage. Again, this may require an ability to understand and utilise pharmacokinetic data. The prescriber should know about common types of medication error and how to prevent them. One major cause of adverse events is incorrect calculation of, for example, dose or rate of administration, both of which have led in the past to patient morbidity and mortality. It is, therefore, vital that the prescriber undertake to develop competence in calculation skills appropriate to performance of the role.

UNITS OF MEASUREMENT

The system of measurement used in the UK is the metric system. In prescribing of medicines, probably the most commonly used units are those of mass and volume. Mass is more commonly referred to as weight and the basic metric unit is the gram (g). The basic metric unit of volume is the litre (L). Drug amounts are also commonly referred to in terms of a base unit called a mole (mol). However, it is common for multiples or fractions of these base units to be used. A competent prescriber should understand what the terms mean and be able to convert between them accurately.

Prefixes

A prefix is a group of letters placed at the beginning of a word that change the meaning of the word. There are three prefixes commonly seen in the UK metric system:

- *kilo*   meaning one thousand times greater than the base unit. For example: a kilogram is 1000 grams

- *milli*   meaning one thousand times less than the base unit. For example: a milligram is 1000th of a gram

- *micro* meaning one million times less than the base unit. For example: a microgram is 1,000,000th of a gram

Units of volume

The base unit of volume is the litre, which is abbreviated either to L or l. The other unit of volume commonly seen is the millilitre abbreviated to ml. One litre is equivalent to 1000 ml. To convert a volume in litres into a volume in ml, we must multiply by 1000. To convert a volume in ml into litres, we must divide by 1000.

Example 1: Convert 1.5 L into ml

$$\text{Volume in ml} = 1.5\,\text{L} \times 1000$$

$$= 1500\,\text{ml}$$

Some people like to think of this as moving the decimal place. To multiply by 1000, you have to move the decimal place three places to the right.

$$1.5 \times 1000 = 1.5\,0\,0$$

$$= 1500\,\text{ml}$$

Example 2: Convert 750 ml into L

$$\text{Volume in L} = \frac{750\,\text{ml}}{1000}$$

$$= 0.75\,\text{L}$$

Some people like to think of this as moving the decimal place. To divide by 1000, you have to move the decimal place three places to the left.

$$\frac{750}{1000} = 7\,5\,0.$$

$$= 0.75\,\text{L}$$

Try these examples:

1. You have a patient who needs some indigestion mixture. The usual dose is 10 ml four times a day. You decide to prescribe enough to last the patient 28 days. Give your answer in litres.

   Step 1: Calculate how much the patient will take in 1 day.

$$10\,\text{ml} \times 4 = 40\,\text{ml}$$

   Step 2: Calculate how much the patient will need for 28 days.

$$40\,\text{ml} \times 28 = 1120\,\text{ml}$$

Step 3: Convert the volume into litres.

$$\frac{1120\,ml}{1000} = 1.12\,L$$

2. You have a patient who needs to be prescribed fluids. The patient needs 35 ml fluid per kilogram body weight per day. He weighs 70 kg. How much fluid will he need? Give your answer in litres.

Step 1: Calculate how much fluid the patient will need in 1 day.

$$35\,ml \times 70 = 2450\,ml$$

Step 2: Convert the volume into litres.

$$\frac{2450\,ml}{1000} = 2.45\,L$$

Units of mass

The base unit of mass, or weight as we commonly say, is the gram, which is abbreviated to g. The other units of mass commonly seen are:

- The kilogram (abbreviated to kg)
- The milligram (abbreviated to mg)
- The microgram

Prescribers should always be very careful to write out 'microgram' *in full* and not to abbreviate it because the abbreviations that have been used (mcg or μg) have sometimes led to drug errors.

The units of mass or weight are related to each other as shown in Table 1.

To convert a weight in kilograms into grams, or a weight of grams into milligrams, or a weight of milligrams into micrograms, we must multiply by 1000.

Example 3: Convert 2.75 kg into g

$$\text{Weight in g} = 2.75\,kg \times 1000$$

$$= 2750\,g$$

Some people like to think of this as moving the decimal place. To multiply by 1000, you have to move the decimal place three places to the right.

Table 12.1   Units of mass

Unit	Abbreviated to	Equivalent to
1 kilogram	kg	1000 g
1 gram	g	1000 mg
1 milligram	mg	1000 micrograms

$$2.75 \times 1000 = 2.7\,5\,0$$
$$= 2750\,g$$

Example 4: Convert 25 g into mg

$$\text{Weight in mg} = 25\,g \times 1000$$
$$= 25{,}000\,mg$$

Example 5: Convert 750 mg into micrograms

$$\text{Weight in microgram} = 750\,mg \times 1000$$
$$= 750{,}000\,micrograms$$

To convert a weight in grams into kilograms, or a weight in mgs into grams, or a weight in micrograms into mgs, we must divide by 1000.

Example 6: Convert 250 micrograms into mg

$$\frac{250}{1000} = 0.25\,mg$$

Some people like to think of this as moving the decimal place. To divide by 1000, you have to move the decimal place three places to the left.

$$\frac{250}{1000} = 2\,5\,0.$$
$$= 0.25\,mg$$

Example 7: Convert 500 mg into g

$$\frac{500\,mg}{1000} = 0.5\,g$$

Example 8: Convert 1400 g into kg

$$\frac{1400}{1000} = 1.4\,kg$$

Try these examples:

1. You need to calculate the daily dose of a drug for a patient. The daily dose is 50 mg per kilogram body weight. Your patient weighs 75 kg. State your answer in grams.

   Step 1: Calculate how much drug the patient will need in 1 day.

   $$50\,mg \times 75 = 3750\,mg$$

   Step 2: Convert the dose into grams.

   $$\frac{3750\,mg}{1000} = 3.75\,g$$

2. The daily dose of immunoglobulin for a patient is 0.4 g per kilogram body weight per day. The patient weighs 70 kg. Calculate the amount needed for a 5-day course. Give your answer in kilograms.

Step 1: Calculate how much drug the patient will need in 1 day.

$$0.4\,g \times 70 = 28\,g$$

Step 2: Calculate how much drug the patient will need for 5 days.

$$28\,g \times 5 = 140\,g$$

Step 3: Convert into kilograms.

$$\frac{140\,g}{1000} = 0.14\,kg$$

3. The dose of medicine for a child is 75 micrograms per kilogram body weight per day. The child weighs 15 kg. Calculate the total daily dose needed by the child in milligrams.

Step 1: Calculate the total daily dose of the drug in microgram.

$$75\ \text{micrograms} \times 15 = 1125\ \text{micrograms}$$

Step 2: Convert the total daily dose into mg.

$$\frac{1125\ \text{micrograms}}{1000} = 1.125\,mg$$

4. A patient needs some cream for eczema. She needs 15 g to apply to her face, 200 g for both arms, 50 g for both hands and 400 g for her trunk. How much do you need to prescribe in total? Give your answer in kg.

Step 1: Add the total amount of cream needed.

Face:	15 g
Both arms:	200 g
Both hands:	50 g
Trunk:	400 g
Total:	665 g

Step 2: Convert the total amount into kg.

$$\frac{665\,g}{1000} = 0.665\,kg$$

Units of amount

The term used for the base unit of the amount of a drug is called a *mole*. We usually see this expressed as a mass or weight. One mole of a substance is the molecular, atomic or ionic weight of the substance expressed in grams. So, for example, one mole of sodium chloride (NaCl) would be the weight of one sodium ion (23) plus the weight of one chloride ion (35.5) expressed in grams, a total of 58.5 g. We often see the term *millimole* (meaning 1000th of a mole) when we look at a patient's biochemistry results. For example, you might see a serum potassium concentration stated as 4 mmol/L.

When we refer to a molar solution, this means that the solution contains one mole of a substance dissolved in 1 L of fluid. So, for example, a molar aqueous solution of NaCl contains 58.5 g in 1 L water. We might use this in looking at intravenous (IV) fluids. 'Normal' saline, or more correctly physiological saline, is NaCl solution 0.9%. This means it contains 0.9 g NaCl in 100 ml, or 9 g in a litre. We can work how many millimoles of Na and Cl are there in a litre of 'normal' saline like this:

Example 9:

One mole of NaCl is 58.5 g

A molar solution of NaCl contains 58.5 g in 1 L

Therefore, a solution containing 9 g NaCl per litre contains:

$$\frac{9}{58.5} \times 1 \text{ mole} = 0.153 \text{ mole}$$

Convert this to millimoles by multiplying by 1000.

$$0.153 \text{ mole} \times 1000 = 153 \text{ mmol}$$

Therefore, 1 L of a 'normal' saline contains 153 mmol Na ions and 153 mmol Cl ions. (In practice, this is commonly rounded down and stated as 150 mmol per litre of Na and of Cl ions).

We will look at percentages and concentrations of solutions in the next section (understanding concentrations).

Test yourself with practice calculations

Before you continue, test yourself with these calculations to make sure you have understood this section. Answers are given at the end of the chapter.

1. Try converting the following amounts:
   a. How much is 1.5 kg in grams?
   b. How much is 37.5 mg in micrograms?
   c. How much is 650 micrograms in milligrams?
   d. How much is 1750 ml in litres?
   e. How much is 0.95 L in millilitres?

2. You have a patient who needs the following amount of ointment for a rash all over her body. Face: 30 g, both hands: 50 g, scalp: 100 g, both arms: 200 g, both legs: 200 g, trunk: 400 g, groin: 25 g. Calculate how much you should prescribe in total. Give your answer in kilograms.

3. The dose of medicine for a child is 150 micrograms per kilogram body weight per day. The child weighs 25 kg. Calculate the total daily dose needed by the child in milligrams.

4. You have a patient who needs to be prescribed fluids. The patient needs 30 ml fluid per kilogram body weight per day. She weighs 65 kg. How much fluid will she need? Give your answer in litres.

5. A patient needs a mixture for indigestion. The dose needed is 20 ml four times a day. How much do you need to prescribe to last for 30 days? Give your answer in litres.

Amount per volume

The usual method of expressing concentration of a liquid preparation that we see is an amount per unit volume. For example, you will see the following:

- micrograms per millilitre expressed as micrograms/ml

- milligrams per millilitre expressed as mg/ml

- millimoles per litre expressed as mmol/L

- grams per litre expressed as g/L

We will need to use this if we are calculating the volume of a solution that we are going to administer to a patient in order to give a specified dose.

Example 1:

If hysocine hydrobromide injection contains 400 micrograms in 1 ml, how would we give a dose of 600 micrograms?

Step 1: Solution contains 400 micrograms in 1 ml solution.

Step 2: The volume of solution that would contain 600 micrograms is:

$$\frac{600}{400} \times 1\,ml = 1.5\,ml$$

Example 2:

If gentamicin injection contains 80 mg in 2 ml, how would we give a dose of 120 mg?

Step 1: Calculate the amount of gentamicin in 1 ml of solution.

Solution contains 80 mg in 2 ml

Therefore, it contains $\frac{80\,mg}{2} = 40\,mg$ in 1 ml

Step 2: Calculate the volume of solution that contains 120 mg gentamicin.

Solution contains 40 mg in 1 ml

Therefore, for a dose of 120 mg, we would need:

$$\frac{120}{40} \times 1\,ml = 3\,ml$$

Example 3:

You need to prescribe a dose of 5 mg/kg of a drug for a child weighing 30 kg. The drug comes as a mixture that contains 100 mg of the drug in 5 ml of solution. What volume of the mixture will contain the right dose?

Step 1: Calculate the total dose of the drug.

$$5\,mg \times 30 = 150\,mg$$

Step 2: Calculate the volume of mixture that contains 150 mg.

Mixture contains 100 mg in 5 ml

Therefore, the volume that contains 150 mg will be:

$$\frac{150}{100} \times 5\,\text{ml} = 7.5\,\text{ml}$$

Example 4:

You need to give a dose of 2 mmol/kg of sodium to a patient weighing 20 kg. You are going to give this using NaCl 30% solution which contains 50 mmol sodium in 10 ml. What volume of NaCl 30% solution will contain the required dose?

Step 1: Calculate the total dose of the drug required.

2 mmol × 20 = 40 mmol

Step 2: Calculate the volume of solution that contains 40 mmol.

Solution contains 50 mmol sodium in 10 ml.

Therefore, the volume that contains 40 mmol will be:

$$\frac{40}{50} \times 10\,\text{ml} = 8\,\text{ml}$$

Percentage concentrations

Some manufacturers express the concentration of their product as a percentage. It is important that we understand what the term percentage means so that we can work out the strength of the product. *A percentage is the amount of ingredient in 100 parts of the product.*

Percentage concentrations can be found in both solid and liquid preparations. You will see the following types of percentage expressions:

% w/v	*This describes a percentage weight in volume.*
	The weight will be in grams and the volume in ml.
	For example: sodium bicarbonate 4.2% w/v solution contains 4.2 g sodium bicarbonate in 100 ml solution.
% w/w	This describes a percentage weight in weight, most commonly of a solid. Both weights will be in grams.
	For example: betamethasone 0.1% w/w cream contains 0.1 g betamethasone in 100 g cream.
% v/v	This describes a percentage volume in volume of a liquid. Both volumes will be in ml.
	For example: liquid paraffin oral emulsion 50% v/v contains 50 ml liquid paraffin in 100 ml emulsion.

Example 5:

How much lidocaine is contained in 5 ml of lidocaine 2% injection?

Step 1: Work out what the percentage strength means in gram per 100 ml.

Lidocaine 2% injection contains 2 g lidocaine in 100 ml solution.

Step 2: Convert the strength of solution to mgs in 100 ml.

$$2 \text{ g in } 100 \text{ ml} = 2 \times 1000 \text{ mg in } 100 \text{ ml}$$
$$= 2000 \text{ mg in } 100 \text{ ml}$$

Step 3: Calculate how much lidocaine there is in 5 ml of the solution.

$$\frac{5}{100} \times 2000 = 100 \text{ mg in 5 ml}$$

Example 6:

How much bupivacaine is contained in 10 ml of bupivacaine 0.5% injection?

Step 1: Work out what the percentage strength means in gram per 100 ml.

Bupivacaine 0.5% injection contains 0.5 g bupivacaine in 100 ml solution.

Step 2: Convert the strength of solution to mg in 100 ml.

$$0.5 \text{ g in } 100 \text{ ml} = 0.5 \times 1000 \text{ mg in } 100 \text{ ml}$$
$$= 500 \text{ mg in } 100 \text{ ml}$$

Step 3: Calculate how much bupivacaine there is in 10 ml of the solution.

$$\frac{10}{100} \times 500 = 50 \text{ mg in 10 ml}$$

Concentrations expressed in ratios or parts

A ratio concentration is often used to describe the concentration of very dilute solutions. It expresses the number of grams of a drug that are dissolved or dispersed in a given number of parts of a solution in ml. For example, adrenaline solution 1 in 1000 contains 1 g adrenaline in 1000 ml of solution. As these solutions tend to be very dilute and yet very potent, we must be particularly careful with these calculations.

Example 7:

How much adrenaline is contained in 1 ml of adrenaline 1 in 1000 solution?

Step 1: Work out what the ratio strength means.

$$\text{Adrenaline 1 in 1000} = 1 \text{ g in 1000 ml}$$

Step 2: Convert the strength of solution to mg.

$$1 \text{ g in } 1000 \text{ ml} = 1 \times 1000 \text{ mg in } 1000 \text{ ml}$$
$$= 1000 \text{ mg in } 1000 \text{ ml}$$

Step 3: Calculate how much adrenaline there is in 1 ml of the solution.

$$\frac{1}{1000} \times 1000 = 1\,mg\;in\;1\,ml$$

Example 8:

How much adrenaline is contained in 10 ml of adrenaline 1 in 10,000 dilute solution?

Step 1: Work out what the ratio strength means.

$$Adrenaline\;1\;in\;10,000 = 1\,g\;in\;10,000\,ml$$

Step 2: Convert the strength of solution to mg.

$$1\,g\;in\;10,000\,ml = 1 \times 1000\,mg\;in\;10,000\,ml$$

$$= 1000\,mg\;in\;10,000\,ml$$

Step 3: Calculate how much adrenaline there is in 10 ml of the solution.

$$\frac{10}{10,000} \times 1000 = 1\,mg\;in\;10\,ml$$

Test yourself with practice calculations

Before you continue, test yourself with these calculations to make sure you have understood this section. Answers are given at the end of the chapter.

6. How much potassium permanganate is contained in 100 ml of potassium permanganate 1 in 10,000 solution?

7. How much hydrogen peroxide is contained in 250 ml of hydrogen peroxide 6% solution?

8. You have levomepromazine injection 25 mg in 1 ml. You want to put a dose of 6.25 mg into a syringe driver. What volume of levomepromazine injection do you need?

9. You want to give a dose of 25 mg per kilogram of a drug to a child weighing 18 kg. The solution you have contains 200 mg in 5 ml. What volume of the solution will contain the right dose?

10. You want to give a bolus dose of 100 mg lidocaine to a patient to control ventricular arrhythmia. The injection solution you have is lidocaine injection 2%. What volume of the injection do you need to give this dose?

CALCULATING THE DOSE

The '*dose*' of a drug is the amount of drug given to the patient to achieve a therapeutic outcome. The calculated dose may be given as a total daily dose in a single administration (such as digoxin 125 micrograms daily) or it may be necessary to divide the dose into smaller amounts given on more than one occasion during the day (such as diclofenac 50 mg three times a day). There are certain patient groups, like children for example, where the need for dose calculation is common. A prescriber must take care to understand clearly statements about dosage and to calculate doses accurately. The dosage statement may, for example, give the amount to be given *per dose* or the amount to be given *in total per day*, which then needs to be divided according to the recommended frequency of administration. The prescriber may also need to round calculated doses up or down in order to match with availability of a drug formulation. For example, for dissolution of gallstones, the dose of ursodeoxycholic acid in the British National Formulary (BNF) is 8–12 mg/kg daily as a single dose at bedtime or in two divided doses (BNF, 2003). For a patient weighing 60 kg, the total daily dose would be 480–720 mg. The product is available as tablets of 150 mg or capsules of 250 mg. Therefore, in order to keep within the required dose range, the prescribed dose would have to be, say 500 mg daily or 250 mg *twice* daily.

Dosage calculations can be based on:

- A given amount of drug per kilogram body weight of the patient.

- A given amount of drug based on a patient's body surface area (BSA).

- A given rate of drug administration per unit time.

Dosage calculations can sometimes be based on a patient's ideal body weight (IBW) rather than actual body weight. The following equations can be used to calculate the IBW (Bonner, 2001).

Male: IBW = (0.9 × height in cm) − 88 kg
Female: IBW = (0.9 × height in cm) − 92 kg

Calculating a dose based on patient's body weight

Try these examples:

Example 1:
Calculate the dose of co-amoxiclav suspension 250/62 for a child aged 7 years weighing 23 kg.

Step 1: Check the recommended dose in the BNF. The stated dose of co-amoxiclav 250/62 for a child aged 6–12 years is 0.4 ml/kg body weight daily given in three divided doses, increased to 0.8 ml/kg body weight in severe infections. We are going to use 0.4 ml/kg/day.

Step 2: Calculate the total daily dose.

$$\text{Daily dose at 0.4 ml/kg} = \text{Patient's weight (kg)} \times \text{Daily dose (ml/kg)}$$

$$= 23\,\text{kg} \times 0.4\,\text{ml/kg/day}$$

$$= 9.2\,\text{ml/day}$$

Step 3: Calculate the dose to be given three times a day.

$$= \frac{9.2\,\text{ml}}{3}$$

$$= 3.07\,\text{ml}$$

Step 4: Convert the dose into a practical dosage for administration to the patient.

A practical dose to prescribe would be 3 ml three times a day.

Example 2:

Calculate the dose of salbutamol oral solution for a child aged 6 months weighing 7.8 kg.

Step 1: Check the recommended dose in the BNF. The stated dose of salbutamol for a child aged 6 months is 100 micrograms/kg body weight four times a day (unlicensed use).

Step 2: Calculate the amount per dose:

Amount per dose at 100 micrograms/kg

$=$ Patient's weight (kg) $\times$ Amount per dose (micrograms/kg)

$=$ 7.8 kg $\times$ 100 micrograms/kg

$=$ 780 micrograms per dose

Step 3: Calculate the volume of salbutamol oral solution that contains 780 micrograms.

Salbutamol oral solution contains 2 mg salbutamol in 5 ml. To make sure we don't mix up the units we should convert this to a strength stated as micrograms in 5 ml.

2 mg in 5 ml $=$ (2 $\times$ 1000 micrograms) in 5 ml

$=$ 2000 micrograms in 5 ml

Therefore, the amount of the oral solution that contains a dose of 780 micrograms would be:

$$\frac{780}{2000} \times 5\,ml = 1.95\,ml$$

Step 4: Convert this dose into a practical dose for administration to the patient.

Oral syringes for children are available in various sizes. It would probably be best to round this dose up to 2 ml. Therefore the dose to prescribe would be 2 ml four times a day of salbutamol oral solution.

Example 3:

Calculate the dose of gentamicin for an adult male patient to treat septicaemia. The dose should be based on IBW as long as the patient's actual weight is greater than this. The patient is 180 cm tall.

Step 1: Check the recommended dose in the BNF. The stated adult dose of gentamicin is 3–5 mg/kg body weight daily given in divided doses every 8 hours. We are going to use 5 mg/kg/day to treat septicaemia.

Step 2: Calculate the patient's IBW.

Male: IBW $=$ (0.9 $\times$ height in cm) $-$ 88 kg

$=$ (0.9 $\times$ 180) $-$ 88 kg

$=$ 74 kg

Step 3: Calculate the total daily dose.

Daily dose at 5 mg/kg = Patient's IBW (kg) × Daily dose (mg/kg)

$$= 74\,kg \times 5\,mg/kg/day$$

$$= 370\,mg/day$$

Step 4: Calculate the dose to be given every 8 hours.

$$= \frac{370\,mg}{3}$$

$$= 123.3\,mg\ per\ dose$$

Step 5: Convert the dose into a practical dosage for administration to the patient.

Gentamicin injection is available in strength of 40 mg in 1 ml.

Therefore a practical dose to prescribe would be 120 mg every 8 hours (three times a day)

Step 6: Calculate the volume of gentamicin injection that contains 120 mg.

If gentamicin injection contains 40 mg in 1 ml, a dose of 120 mg would be equivalent to:

$$\frac{120}{40} \times 1\,ml = 3\,ml$$

The dose of gentamicin based on IBW weight would therefore be 120 mg (3 ml) every 8 hours of gentamicin injection 40 mg in 1 ml.

Calculating a dose for a child as a proportion of the adult dose

With the advent of drug formularies produced especially for children, it is less common to calculate a dose as a proportion of the adult dose. However, examples can still be found in the BNF (BNF, 2003).

Example 1: Oral administration of flucloxacillin

The oral dose of flucloxacillin for a child is stated in the BNF as:

For a child aged less than 2 years: quarter of adult dose

For a child aged 2–10 years: half adult dose

Adult dose is 250–500 mg qds

To calculate a quarter of the adult dose for a child less than 2 years old:

$$250\,mg \times \frac{1}{4} = 62.5\,mg$$

$$500\,mg \times \frac{1}{4} = 125\,mg$$

To calculate a half of the adult dose for a child aged 2–10 years:

$$250\,mg \times \frac{1}{2} = 125\,mg$$

$$500\,mg \times \frac{1}{2} = 250\,mg$$

Calculating the dose based on a patient's BSA

Some dosage calculations are based on the patient's BSA as opposed to body weight. BSA calculations were originally introduced to work out safe starting doses in the early stages of trials of drugs in humans that had previously only been tested in animals. It has become routine practice for dosing of many anti-cancer drugs, although response (or toxicity) is not always closely related to BSA. Calculations used in adult oncology were originally constructed from a study by DuBois and DuBois (1916). This study utilised only nine patients and its accuracy has been disputed (Du Bois, 1916; Wang, 1992). However, because the method is still widely used, prescribers involved in oncology will need to be able to calculate the dosage of drugs using this method.

In general, BSA is estimated using a nomogram. Prescribers must be careful to select the correct nomogram because different ones are available for adults and children. Prescribing in oncology is a specialised and high-risk field of practice. These calculation examples are merely included to raise awareness of this method of calculating doses. Anyone anticipating working in the field of oncology must ensure that further specialist training in dosage calculation is undertaken.

Example 1:
Calculate the dose of cyclophosphamide using the low-dose IV regimen for an adult patient with a BSA estimated at $2.2\,m^2$.

Step 1: Check the recommended dose in the manufacturer's Summary of Product Characteristics for cyclophosphamide. This is stated as follows:

Low dose: $80–240\,mg/m^2$ as a single dose weekly intravenously.

Say we chose $80\,mg/m^2$

Step 2: Calculate the dose for a patient with a BSA of $2.2\,m^2$.

$$Weekly\ dose = 80\,mg/m^2 \times 2.2\,m^2$$
$$= 176\,mg$$

In general, doses of cytotoxic drugs are not rounded up or down but are prepared individually for the patient.

Example 2:
Calculate the IV dose of vincristine for a child with a BSA estimated at $0.6\,m^2$.

Step 1: Check the recommended dose in the manufacturer's Summary of Product Characteristics for vincristine (Medicines Compendium, 2003a). This is stated as follows:

Children: the usual weekly dose is $2\,mg/m^2$

Step 2: Calculate the dose for a child with a BSA of $0.6\,m^2$.

$$Weekly\ IV\ dose = 2\,mg/m^2 \times 0.6\,m^2$$
$$= 1.2\,mg$$

Test yourself with practice calculations

Before you continue, test yourself with these calculations to make sure you have understood this section. Answers are given at the end of the chapter.

11. What is the IBW of the following patients?
    A man who is 185 cm tall?
    A woman who is 150 cm tall?

12. What is the dose of co-amoxiclav suspension 125/35 for a child aged 3 years weighing 16 kg? (use the dose stated in ml/kg body weight from your Nurse Prescribers' Formulary (NPF))

13. Calculate the dose of tobramycin for an adult female to treat a severe infection to be given by slow IV bolus injection. The dose recommended in the BNF is 3 mg/kg daily in divided doses every 8 hours. The dose must be based on IBW. The patient is 165 cm tall.

14. Calculate the dose of cyclophosphamide using the low-dose IV regimen for an adult patient with a BSA estimated at 1.95 m^2. The selected dose is 120 mg/m^2 once a week.

CALCULATING THE RATE OF DRUG ADMINISTRATION PER UNIT TIME

There are many occasions when drugs are administered by infusion. Possible routes of administration include IV, subcutaneous and epidural. Infusions have a high-risk potential for patients, partially because they may involve the administration of large volumes of fluid, and partially because the drugs given by infusion tend to be very potent. This is another area where calculation skills are important. Although nurse prescribers may not be involved in prescribing these types of infusion under current legislation, with the possible exception of those working in palliative care, they should be competent to check correctly their colleagues undertaking such a procedure, either prescribing or administration.

Calculating the rate of administration of an infusion to be given using a volumetric infusion device set in drops per minute

Volumetric giving sets are often used to administer large volumes of IV fluid to patients. Although not particularly accurate, it is possible to calculate the rate of administration such that a certain volume will be delivered to a patient over the required time. For the purposes of this chapter, we will assume that an adult volumetric giving set administers 1 ml of for every 20 drops of solution.

Care: *This may be different for blood giving sets and for paediatric giving sets. Always check the number of drops per ml for the particular giving set you are using.*

Example 1:

Say you wanted to administer 1 L of glucose 5% infusion over 8 h.

Step 1: Convert the volume of solution into ml.

$$1 \text{ L over } 8 \text{ h} = 1000 \text{ ml over } 8 \text{ h}$$

Step 2: Calculate the volume of solution to be given per hour.

$$1000 \text{ ml over } 8 \text{ h} = \frac{1000 \text{ ml}}{8} = 125 \text{ ml/h}$$

Step 3: Calculate the volume of solution to be given per minute.

$$125\,\text{ml over 1h} = \frac{125}{60} = 2.08\,\text{ml/min}$$

This could be rounded down to 2 ml per minute as this method of administration is not accurate to two decimal places.

Step 4: Calculate the number of drops equivalent to this volume.

Using our chosen giving set, we must administer 20 drops to give 1 ml solution.

Therefore 2 ml = 40 drops.

Therefore the drip controller should be set so that it administers 40 drops in one minute in order to administer 1 L of fluid over 8 hours.

Calculating the rate of administration of an infusion to be given using a high-risk infusion device set in ml per hour

Administration of drugs by the IV route is a high-risk procedure. Hospital pharmacists generally try to help make this procedure safer by producing monographs for IV administration. Often, for high-risk drugs such as dopamine, a standard table of administration according to required rate of administration and patient's weight will be available. However, health professionals should be aware of how such tables are calculated.

Before administering a drug intravenously, the nurse should check:

- That the situation of the patient matches the monograph. For example, some drugs can only be given in critical care areas with appropriate close monitoring of the patient. The IV monograph may specify a critical care area with certain patient monitoring facilities.
- That the drug can be given through the available IV line. For example, some drugs can be given only via a central line because they are highly acidic or alkaline and would damage a peripheral vein where the blood flow is slower.
- That the drug can be given through the available IV line in the concentration prescribed. For example, the concentration of some drug solutions varies according to whether a central or peripheral line is used. The monograph provided should specify this.
- That the patient details correspond with the types of patient mentioned in the monograph. For example, there will be different monographs for adults, children and neonates.
- That the dose to be administered is appropriate. The monograph will normally include a statement of the correct dose to be administered according to the indication for the drug.
- That the prescribed diluent is correct. Some drugs can only be diluted in certain diluents. For example, amiodarone can only be given in glucose 5% solution.

Example 2:

Calculate the rate of administration in ml per hour of dopamine infusion for a patient weighing 60 kg. The dopamine infusion is to go through a peripheral line at a rate of

3 micrograms/kg/minute diluted in normal saline. The recommended dilution of the infusion for peripheral administration is 800 mg dopamine in 500 ml normal saline.

Step 1: Calculate the dose in microgram/min for a 60 kg patient.

Dopamine is to be given at a rate of 3 micrograms/kg/min. Patient weighs 60 kg.

$$3 \text{ micrograms/kg/min} \times 60 \text{ kg} = 180 \text{ micrograms/min}$$

Step 2: Calculate the dose in microgram/hour for a 60 kg patient.

$$180 \text{ micrograms/min} \times 60 \text{ min} = 10{,}800 \text{ micrograms/h}$$

Step 3: Convert the dose into mg/h.

$$1 \text{ mg} = 1000 \text{ micrograms}$$

$$\text{Therefore } 10{,}800 \text{ micrograms} = 10.8 \text{ mg/h}$$

Step 4: Check the recommended dilution of the solution for the infusion method selected.

The recommended dilution of the infusion for peripheral administration is 800 mg dopamine in 500 ml normal saline.

Step 5: Convert the calculated dose into a practical dose for administration. In other words, what would be the rate of administration in ml/h to achieve a rate of 10.8 mg/h?

If a solution contains 800 mg in 500 ml, how much does it contain in 1 ml?

$$\frac{1 \text{ ml}}{500 \text{ ml}} \times 800 \text{ mg} = 1.6 \text{ mg in 1 ml}$$

Therefore, how much of the solution would contain 10.8 mg?

$$\frac{10.8}{1.6 \text{ mg}} \times 1 \text{ ml} = 6.75 \text{ ml}$$

Therefore, the rate of administration in ml per hour to achieve a rate of administration of 10.8 mg/h would be 6.75 ml/h.

Example 3:

Calculate the dose of aminophylline to treat an adult with an acute severe asthma attack. Assume that the patient has not previously been treated with theophylline or aminophylline.

The patient weighs 85 kg. You need to give a loading dose of 5 mg per kg given over 20 minutes then a maintenance dose of 500 micrograms/kg/hr. The solution of aminophylline is made up as 500 mg in 500 ml of either normal saline or glucose 5% solution.

Step 1: Calculate the loading dose.

$$5 \text{ mg/kg} \times 85 \text{ kg} = 425 \text{ mg over 20 mins in either normal saline}$$
$$\text{or glucose 5\% infusion.}$$

Step 2: Calculate the maintenance dose.

$$500 \text{ micrograms/kg/h in a patient weighing } 85 \text{ kg} = 500 \times 85 \text{ micrograms/h}$$
$$= 42{,}500 \text{ micrograms/h}$$

Step 3: Convert to mg/hour.

$$42{,}500 \text{ micrograms/h} = \frac{42{,}500}{1000} \text{ mg/h}$$
$$= 42.5 \text{ mg/h}$$

Step 4: Calculate the rate of administration.

The solution contains 500 mg in 500 ml, or 1 mg in 1 ml.

Therefore the maintenance infusion should be set at 42.5 ml/h.

Test yourself with practice calculations

15. A patient requires 1 L of normal saline to be given over 12 h. What is the correct rate for the drip controller in drops per minute assuming the giving set delivers 20 drops for 1 ml of solution?

16. A patient requires 500 ml glucose 5% to be given over 3 h. What is the correct rate for the drip controller in drops per minute assuming the giving set delivers 20 drops for 1 ml of solution?

17. Calculate the rate of administration in millilitres per hour of dobutamine infusion to be administered at a rate of 2.5 micrograms/kg/min to a patient weighing 75 kg. The solution should be made up (according to the IV monograph for critical care areas) as dobutamine 250 mg in 500 ml NaCl 0.9% infusion.

18. Calculate the rate of administration in ml/h of dopamine infusion to be administered at a rate of 2 micrograms/kg/min to a patient weighing 65 kg. The solution will be made up as dopamine 800 mg in 500 ml NaCl 0.9% solution (normal saline).

19. Calculate the dose of aminophylline infusion to treat an adult with an acute severe asthma attack. Assume that the patient has not previously been treated with theophylline or aminophylline.

    The patient weighs 65 kg. You need to prescribe a loading dose of 5 mg per kg given over 20 min then a maintenance dose of 500 micrograms/kg/h. The solution of aminophylline is made up as 500 mg in 500 ml.

CALCULATING UNIT COSTS OF DRUGS

One of the competencies for supplementary (SP) and independent prescribers (IPs) is to prescribe in a cost-effective way. There is a science which looks at cost-effectiveness and clinical effectiveness of drugs called pharmacoeconomics. We are not trying to look at this topic in the amount of detail needed for a full pharmacoeconomic analysis. Here, we will be looking at a way of calculating the cost of treatment courses of drugs so that a simple cost comparison may be made.

Example 1:
a. How to work out the cost of a medicine per day.

What information do you need?

Cost per pack

Number of dose units in the pack

Number of dose units used per day

Example: Cimetidine tablets 400 mg

Cost per pack = £5.58 (current BNF price)

Number of tablets in a pack = 60

Daily dose: 2 tablets/day

You may find it easier to convert the cost of the pack into pence here so that you know the answer will be in pence.

Calculate the cost per tablet:

$$60 \text{ tablets} = £5.58 = 558 \text{ pence}$$

$$1 \text{ tablet} = \frac{558}{60} = 9 \text{ pence}$$

Calculate the cost per day:

$$9 \text{ pence/tablet} \times 2 \text{ tablets/day} = 18 \text{ pence/day}$$

b. How to work out the cost per treatment course?

What information do you need?

Cost per day

Number of weeks or days in the course

Example: Cimetidine tablets 400 mg

Cost/day = 18 pence

Number of weeks in the course = 8 weeks

Therefore number of days in the course = $8 \times 7 = 56$ days

Calculate the cost per course:

$$18 \text{ pence/day} \times 56 \text{ days} = 1008 \text{ pence} = £10.08$$

In the real situation, if you wanted to compare cimetidine with other histamine H_2 antagonists, you would also need to consider how long was the treatment course for each drug, what percentage of patients were cured by the standard treatment course, what were the comparative relapse rates etc. However, this method would enable you to compare different treatment regimes in terms of drug cost alone.

Test yourself with practice calculations

20. Calculate the comparative monthly treatment costs of the following non-steroidal anti-inflammatory drugs (NSAIDs).

Drug	Pack size	Cost per pack (£)	Treatment course (days)	Daily dose (mg tds)
Ibuprofen tablets 400 mg	84	2.46	28	400
Diclofenac tablets 50 mg	84	3.67	28	50
Naproxen tablets 500 mg	28	3.08	28	500

21. Calculate the monthly treatment costs of the following antacids assuming they are taken regularly in the dose listed in the table, in each case the upper end of the recommended dosage range.

Drug	Pack size (ml)	Cost per pack (£)	Treatment course (days)	Daily dose (ml qds)
Algicon susp	500	3.07	28	20
Gastrocote liq	500	2.67	28	15
Gaviscon liq	500	2.70	28	20
Gaviscon advance liq	500	6.44	28	10

SIMPLE PHARMACOKINETIC CALCULATIONS

Pharmacokinetics is a topic included within the core curriculum for independent and supplementary prescribing. Pharmacokinetic calculations can be very complex and you may need a specialist practitioner, such as a clinical pharmacist, to help you with them. However, some simple calculations can help you when you are counselling your patients on their medication. They can also help when you are converting between routes of administration of a drug.

Half-life

The half-life of a drug is the time taken for the plasma concentration of the drug to reduce by half. It is relatively constant for a given drug, assuming no change in the patient's liver or renal function, although in some cases there may be wide inter-patient variation. So why is half-life important?

When a patient starts taking a drug and continues to take it regularly at the prescribed intervals, the blood level of the drug gradually increases until it becomes constant. This constant blood level is called the 'steady state plasma concentration'. For a drug with a simple pharmacokinetic profile, although it may begin to take effect after the first dose, it will generally not reach its full effect until steady state plasma concentration is reached. This will be after four to five times the half-life of a drug. Table 12.2 shows you why this is the case.

The patient is given a dose at time zero and it will achieve a certain blood level. After one half-life, the blood level will have fallen to half its original value, say

Table 12.2 Plasma concentration after repeated oral dosing of a drug (where the dose interval is the same as the half-life)

Number of half-lives	Number of doses	Plasma concentration remaining from each dose (mg/L)						Total plasma concentration (mg/L)
1	1	10.00						10.00
2	2	5.00	10.00					15.00
3	3	2.50	5.00	10.00				17.50
4	4	1.25	2.50	5.00	10.00			18.75
5	5	0.625	1.25	2.50	5.00	10.00		19.38
6	6	0.3125	0.625	1.25	2.50	5.00	10.00	19.69

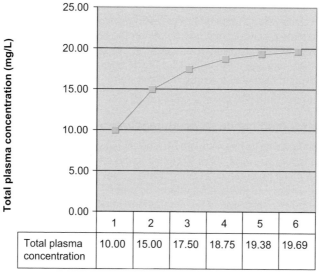

	1	2	3	4	5	6
Total plasma concentration	10.00	15.00	17.50	18.75	19.38	19.69

Number of half-lives

Figure 12.1 Increasing total plasma concentration with number of half-lives at the beginning of dosing

10 mg/L, as the drug is excreted. After a second half-life it will fall by half again to 5 mg/L. After a third half-life it will fall by half again to 2.5 mg/L and so on. But say we give more doses. Each dose will achieve the original blood level and start falling off as it is excreted. Each time a dose is given, a portion of that dose will be retained at each half-life. All of these portions together add up to make the total blood level (or total plasma concentration). We can see from the Figure 12.1 that

Table 12.3   Plasma concentration at the end of dosing of a drug

Number of half-lives	Total plasma concentration (mg/L)
0	20.00
1	10.00
2	5.00
3	2.50
4	1.25
5	0.625

the plasma concentration starts to flatten out at around five half-lives and this is called 'steady state plasma concentration'.

The reverse is true when the patient stops taking a drug. The initial blood level will be the steady state plasma concentration. When the patient stops taking the drug, the blood level will fall to half of its original concentration at each half-life. Therefore, as we can see from Table 12.3, it will take about four to five times the half-life of a drug to eliminate the drug from the body.

Understanding the term half-life of a drug is important for various reasons:

Time taken for medication to reach maximum effect

Consider ibuprofen with its half-life of about 2 hours (Davis, 2001). If a patient started taking ibuprofen for pain relief, there would be some effect from the first dose when it reached the initial peak plasma concentration after about an hour. However, in order to obtain maximum therapeutic effect, the patient would need to continue taking the drug regularly according to the recommended dosing schedule. Steady state plasma concentration, and thus maximum pain relief, would be reached after about 8–10 hours (four to five times the half-life of 2 hours). Patient confidence in the prescriber is likely to be increased if this type of information can be given.

Example 1:

Naproxen is a NSAID with a half-life of about 14 hours (Davis, 2001). If you prescribed this drug and the patient took it regularly according to the recommended dosing schedule, how long would it take to reach steady state plasma concentration?

Step 1: Earliest time to steady state plasma concentration.

$$= 4 \times 14\,h$$

$$= 56\,h$$

Step 2: Longest time to steady state plasma concentration.

$$= 5 \times 14\,h$$

$$= 70\,h$$

Time for the effect of medication to wear off

Some drugs have a very long half-life. If a patient was getting side-effects and the decision was taken to discontinue the drug, it would take 4–5 half-lives for the drug to be eliminated and for its effect to wear off completely. For example, if a patient was taking digoxin, with a half-life of about 40 h (Bauman, 2001) (assuming normal renal function), it would take over a week to eliminate digoxin from the blood stream. Any toxic effects would wear off sometime during that week as the blood level fell.

Example 2:

A patient was taking digoxin but was getting toxic effects including nausea and diarrhoea. A blood level was reported as 2.8 nanograms/ml. If the patient stopped taking digoxin, how long would it take for the blood level to fall to 0.35 nanograms/ml? Assume that the half-life of digoxin in this patient is 40 h.

Step 1: After one half-life (40 h), the digoxin level will have reduced by half.

$$\frac{2.8 \text{ nanograms/ml}}{2} = 1.4 \text{ nanograms/ml}$$

Step 2: After a second half-life (40 h), the digoxin level will have reduced by half again.

$$\frac{1.4 \text{ nanograms/ml}}{2} = 0.7 \text{ nanograms/ml}$$

Step 3: After a third half-life (40 h), the digoxin level will have reduced by half again.

$$\frac{0.7 \text{ nanograms/ml}}{2} = 0.35 \text{ nanograms/ml}$$

Step 4: Therefore the digoxin level will fall to 0.35 nanograms/ml after $3 \times$ half-life

$$= 3 \times 40 \text{ h} = 120 \text{ h}.$$

Change of half-life depending on the patient

The half-life of a drug is relatively constant in a given patient group but it can vary between different patient groups. For example, because digoxin is renally excreted, its half-life is extended in patients with poor renal function, up to 4–5 days (Bauman, 2001). Some drugs have a different half-life in children because of their different body composition and systems for eliminating drugs. Gentamicin, for example has a half-life of about 2 h in a normal adult, but about 3 h in an older infant, or about 50–70 h in an adult patient with anuria (Flaherty, 2001a).

This information about half-life is something of a generalisation because of the following:

- The clinical effect of some drugs is not directly related to the plasma concentration. Tricyclic antidepressants used to treat depression and disease-modifying drugs used to treat rheumatoid arthritis are two examples of drugs known to take a few weeks to take effect.

- Some drugs are metabolised to produce active metabolites. These metabolites will have their own half-lives. The effect of the drug may be related to the half-life of the metabolite(s), not just the drug itself. For example, the serum level of chlorpheniramine does not correlate with its histamine antagonist activity because of an active metabolite (Ashton, 2001).

- Genetic differences between patients can mean that there is wide inter-patient variation in steady state plasma levels. For example, there can be a 30-fold variation in steady state plasma level between patients taking the same dose of heterocyclic antidepressants (Stimmel, 2001).

Bioavailability

Bioavailability of a drug is the fraction of the dose administered that reaches the systemic circulation. It estimates the extent but not the rate of absorption. For an IV injection, the bioavailability is 100% because all of the dose is put directly into the systemic circulation. If a drug is given by another route of administration, then less than 100% of the drug may reach the blood stream. This may be due to a variety of causes such as extensive metabolism of the drug in the liver, the relative lipid and water solubility of the drug molecule that determines whether it will cross cell membranes, breakdown of the drug in the gastrointestinal tract and many other factors. It is not possible to administer some drugs orally because the amount of drug reaching the systemic circulation via this route is negligible.

Once a drug has been marketed, the manufacturer will have designed a dosage form that will allow sufficient drug into the blood stream to have the required clinical effect. However, it is important to know about relative bioavailability of different dosage forms of the same drug to determine of a dosage change is required when the route of administration is changed. A good example of this would be benzylpenicillin (penicillin G). When given intravenously, 100% of the injection reaches the blood stream. However, when given orally only 15–30% of the drug is absorbed because the drug is broken down by acid in the stomach. It is common to give penicillin V if the oral route is required because this has more complete (60%) and more reliable oral absorption (Flaherty, 2001b).

A knowledge of bioavailability is important if changing from one route of administration to another. Here are some examples:

- Carbamazepine can be given by mouth to treat, amongst other things, epilepsy. If the patient is unable to take medication by the oral route, suppositories are available but a dose of 100 mg orally is equivalent to a dose of 125 mg rectally (BNF, 2003). An additional problem is that absorption from carbamazepine suppositories is saturable and the maximum dose to be given per dose is 250 mg. Therefore a change of dosage frequency may also be needed.

Example 1:

A patient has been stabilised on an oral dose of carbamazepine of 300 mg twice a day. What is the equivalent dose in suppositories?

Step 1: Total daily dose of carbamazepine $= 300\,mg \times 2 = 600\,mg$.

Step 2: Convert 600 mg orally to the equivalent in suppositories.

$$100\,mg \text{ orally} = 125\,mg \text{ rectally}$$

$$\text{Therefore, } 600\,mg \text{ orally} = (6 \times 125\,mg) \text{ rectally}$$

$$= 750\,mg$$

Step 3: Not more than 250 mg can be given at a time by the rectal route. Therefore a rectal dose of 750 mg must be given as 250 mg three times a day.

- Sodium fucidate tablets are given by mouth to treat staphylococcal infections. The usual adult dose of the tablets is 500 mg three times a day. If the patient requires a liquid preparation, the suspension contains fusidic acid which is less completely absorbed. The usual adult dose of the suspension is 750 mg three times a day (BNF, 2003).

- Phenytoin sodium, another anti-epileptic drug, is given by mouth in capsule form commonly in a dose of 150–300 mg daily. If the patient requires a liquid preparation, the suspension contains phenytoin base. The conversion recommended in the BNF is that phenytoin sodium 100 mg (capsule) is equivalent therapeutically to phenytoin 90 mg (suspension or liquid) (Davis, 2001).

Example 2:

A patient has been stabilised on an oral dose of phenytoin sodium capsules of 300 mg daily. What is the equivalent dose of phenytoin liquid?

Step 1: Phenytoin sodium capsule 100 mg = phenytoin liquid 90 mg.

Step 2: Phenytoin sodium capsule (3 × 100 mg)

$$= \text{phenytoin liquid } (3 \times 90 \text{ mg})$$

$$= \text{phenytoin liquid } 270 \text{ mg}$$

Step 3: Phenytoin liquid contains 30 mg phenytoin in 5 ml. Therefore what volume contains 270 mg?

$$\frac{270 \text{ mg}}{30 \text{ mg}} \times 5 \text{ ml} = 45 \text{ ml}$$

Test yourself with practice calculations

Before you continue, test yourself with these calculations to make sure you have understood this section. Answers are given at the end of the chapter.

22. What is the time to steady state plasma concentration of the following drugs? Assume that steady state is reached after five half-lives and that the drug is taken regularly by the patient.

Drug	Half-life (h)
Paracetamol	2
Indomethacin	2.4
Meloxicam	20
Piroxicam	48

From: Davis, 2001.

23. A patient has been taking theophylline and has a toxic plasma level of 28 mg/L. The half-life of theophylline in this patient is estimated as 8 h. How long would it take for the plasma concentration to fall within reference range for theophylline (10–15 mg/L)?

24. You have an epileptic patient who has been taking phenytoin sodium capsules 350 mg daily for several weeks and is well controlled. However, she has had a stroke and can no longer swallow the capsules. What is the equivalent dose of phenytoin suspension?

25. You have an epileptic patient who has been taking carbamazepine 400 mg twice daily orally for several weeks and is well controlled. However, she is nil-by-mouth at the moment. What is the equivalent dose in suppositories?

PALLIATIVE CARE

Syringe drivers

In palliative care, patients often receive drugs via a syringe driver. The legislation surrounding prescribing of controlled drugs is constantly changing with respect to independent nurse prescribing, patient group directions and supplementary prescribing. Prescribers must make sure they are aware of the current legislation using an up-to-date source such as the Department of Health (DoH) website (http://www.dh.gov.uk/Home/fs/en) or Nurse Prescriber website (http://www.nurse-prescriber.co.uk).

Caution: *when drugs are combined in a syringe driver, this is off-licence prescribing. The prescriber assumes liability for the final product. Compatibility of the resulting solution must always be checked using a specialist medicines information source such as a palliative care handbook. Compatibility will depend on:*

- *The drug combination used*
- *The diluent used to make up the solution*
- *The final concentration of each ingredient in the solution*

Prescribers should be aware of how to calculate the ingredients in a syringe driver in the event that they make up the device content for administration to the patient and also, so that appropriate quantities of injection solutions can be prescribed.

We have already looked at how to calculate the volume of injection containing a given dose of medication. Here is a reminder:

Example 1:
If metoclopramide injection contains 10 mg in 1 ml, what volume contains 15 mg?

$$\frac{15}{10} \times 1 = 1.5\,\text{ml}$$

Example 2:
If hyoscine hydrobromide injection contains 400 micrograms in 1 ml, what volume contains 300 micrograms?

$$\frac{300}{400} \times 1 = 0.75\,\text{ml}$$

In order to calculate the content of a syringe driver, we must calculate the volume of each injection solution to be added. We must also know the final volume of the syringe driver we are intending to make up so that we can work out how much diluent we need.

Example 3:

If we wanted to make up a syringe driver to contain diamorphine 10 mg (reconstituted with 1 ml water for injection) and cyclizine 50 mg (1 ml) and the final volume of the syringe driver was 10 ml, the amount of water for injection that would be required is 10 ml − 1 ml − 1 ml = 8 ml. Therefore the prescriber would need to ensure the patient had a supply of 10 ml vials of water for injection to be able to make up the final volume.

Calculation of breakthrough analgesia doses

If morphine is being given in the form of slow-release tablets, patients are usually prescribed a dose of non-slow-release morphine to take when needed for breakthrough pain. Non-slow-release morphine acts for about 4 h and is therefore usually given up to six times a day. This is used to provide a formula for calculating how big the breakthrough dose should be:

$$\text{Breakthrough dose} = \frac{\text{(total daily dose of slow-release morphine)}}{6}$$

Example 1:

If a patient is taking morphine sulphate slow-release tablets 120 mg twice a day, what should the breakthrough dose of non-slow-release morphine be?

Step 1: Total daily dose of slow-release morphine = 120 mg × 2 = 240 mg

Step 2: Breakthrough dose of non-slow-release morphine is:

$$\frac{240 \text{ mg}}{6} = 40 \text{ mg}$$

A dose of 40 mg non-slow-release morphine should be prescribed to be taken when required for breakthrough pain.

Changing from oral morphine to diamorphine injection

When patients are first changed over to a syringe driver, they will usually have been taking oral morphine beforehand. There is a table with suggested dosage conversion in the NPF. The approximate dose conversion is usually taken as:

3 mg oral morphine = 1 mg sub-cutaneous diamorphine

This may vary according to the reference text used. Some authors allow for the fact that starting a syringe driver usually indicates loss of control of pain and an automatic slight increase in dose is built in. When calculating the total dose of oral morphine, we must remember to add the total of the non-slow-release doses used for breakthrough pain as well as the regular slow-release doses.

Example 2:

We will use the 3:1 ratio for our example. A patient is taking morphine sulphate slow-release tablets 100 mg twice a day for pain and morphine sulphate non-slow-release tablets 30 mg about four times a day for breakthrough pain. You want to change to a syringe driver. What is the equivalent sub-cutaneous dose of diamorphine?

Step 1: Calculate the total daily dose of oral morphine:

Slow-release morphine: 100 mg twice a day = 200 mg

Non-slow-release morphine: 30 mg four times a day = 120 mg

Total daily dose of morphine = 320 mg

Step 2: Calculate the equivalent sub-cutaneous dose of diamorphine.

3 mg oral morphine = 1 mg sub-cutaneous diamorphine

Therefore a dose of 320 mg oral morphine is equivalent to:

$$320 \times \frac{1}{3} = 106.7\,mg$$

Step 3: Round this dose to a suitable dose for the patient.

In practice it would not be practical to give a dose of 106.7 mg of diamorphine. Therefore, the dose would be rounded up to 110 mg or down to 100 mg according to the patient's needs.

Changing from oral morphine to fentanyl patch

Fentanyl patches are a slow-release dosage form providing opiate analgesia at a steady rate over 3 days. Patients are often converted from oral morphine to fentanyl patches as they may provide a more constant level of analgesia. When converting, the following formula is used (ref. NPF section 4.7.2).

Oral morphine sulphate 90 mg in 24 h = fentanyl patch 25 micrograms/h.

Example 1:

If a patient was taking morphine sulphate slow-release 90 mg twice a day, the equivalent dose of fentanyl patch would be:

90 mg × 2 = 180 mg/day = fentanyl patch 50 micrograms/h

As the patches are only available in 25, 50, 75 and 100 microgram strengths, this dose conversion requires an amount of dose banding and the manufacturer provides a dosage conversion table in the SPC (Medicines Compendium 2003b).

Test yourself with practice calculations

26. Calculate the contents of the following syringe driver in ml.

Diamorphine hydrochloride 50 mg (dissolved in 2 ml water for injection)
Metoclopramide 40 mg
Levomepromazine 12.5 mg
Water for injection to 17 ml

Oral 24 hour morphine (mg/day)	Fentanyl patch (micrograms/h)
<135	25
135–224	50
225–314	75
315–404	100
405–494	125
495–584	150
585–674	175
675–764	200
765–854	225
855–944	250
945–1034	275
1035–1124	300

This formulation has been checked for stability (Dickman, 2002).

27. A patient is taking 60 mg morphine sulphate slow-release tablets twice a day. What is the correct dose of oral morphine sulphate solution for breakthrough pain?

28. A patient is taking 15 mg of morphine sulphate solution every 4 h regularly. What is the equivalent dose of slow-release morphine tablets to be taken every 12 h?

29. A patient is taking 120 mg morphine sulphate slow-release tablets bd. Calculate the equivalent dose of fentanyl patches. Remember that you may need to round up or round down to the nearest whole patch. Check your answer using the table provided.

30. A patient is taking 90 mg morphine sulphate slow-release tablets bd regularly and is needing about 4 × 30 mg breakthrough doses of oral morphine solution. Calculate the equivalent dose of diamorphine to use if the patient was converted to a syringe driver.

References

Ashton L (2001). Antihistamines. In: *Handbook of Clinical Drug Data*, 10th edn (Anderson P, Knoben J, Troutman W). Stamford, Connecticut: Appleton and Lange.

Bauman J (2001). Antiarrhythmic Drugs. In: *Handbook of Clinical Drug Data*, 10th edn (Anderson P, Knoben J, Troutman W). Stamford, Connecticut: Appleton and Lange.

Bonner M, Wright D, George B (2001). *Practical Pharmaceutical Calculations*. Newbury: Petroc Press (LibraPharm Limited).

British National Formulary 46 (September 2003). British Medical Association and Royal Pharmaceutical Society of Great Britain.

Davis L J (2001). Nonsteroidal Anti-inflammatory Drugs. In: *Handbook of Clinical Drug Data*, 10th edn (Anderson P, Knoben J, Troutman W). Stamford Connecticut: Appleton and Lange.

Dickman A, Littlewood C, Varga J (2002). *The Syringe Driver. Subcutaneous Infusions in Palliative Care*. Oxford: Oxford University Press.

DuBois and DuBois (1916). Cited in Jones PR, Wilkinson S, Davies PS (1985). A revision of body surface area estimations, *European Journal of Applied Physiology and Occupational Physiology* **53(4)**: 376–379.

Flaherty J (2001a). Aminoglycosides. In: *Handbook of Clinical Drug Data*, 10th edn (Anderson P, Knoben J, Troutman W). Stamford, Connecticut: Appleton and Lange.

Flaherty J (2001b). Beta-lactams. In: *Handbook of Clinical Drug Data*, 10th edn. (Anderson P, Knoben J, Troutman W). Stamford, Connecticut: Appleton and Lange.

Medicines Compendium (2003a). *Summary of Product Characteristics. Oncovin*. Eli Lilly and Co Ltd: p. 1578. http://emc.medicines.org.uk.

Medicines Compendium (2003b). *Summary of Product Characteristics. Durogesic*. Janssen-Cilag Ltd. p. 648. http://emc.medicines.org.uk.

NPC (November 2001). *Maintaining Competency in Prescribing: An Outline Framework to Help Nurse Prescribers*. http://www.npc.co.uk/nurse_prescribing/pdfs/maint_comp_in_prescrib.pdf.

NPC (March 2003). *Maintaining Competency in Prescribing: An Outline Framework to Help Pharmacist Supplementary Prescribers*. http://www.npc.co.uk/publications/maint_compt_presc/supplementary_red.pdf.

Stimmel G (2001). Antidepressants. In: *Handbook of Clinical Drug Data*, 10th edn (Anderson P, Knoben J, Troutman W). Stamford, Connecticut: Appleton and Lange.

Wang Y, Moss J, Thisted R (1992). Predictors of body surface area. *Journal of Clinical Anesthesia* **4(1)**: 4–10.

CALCULATION SKILLS

Answers

1. (a) 1.5 kg × 1000   = 1500 g
   (b) 37.5 mg × 1000   = 37,500 micrograms
   (c) 650 microgram/1000 = 0.65 mg
   (d) 1750 ml/1000   = 1.75 L
   (e) 0.95 L × 1000   = 950 ml

2. Total amount of ointment:
   Face: 30 g
   Both hands: 50 g
   Scalp: 100 g
   Both arms: 200 g
   Both legs: 200 g

Trunk: 400 g
Groin: 25 g
Total: 1005 g

$$\text{Total amount in kg is } \frac{1005}{1000} = 1.005 \, kg$$

3. Calculate the total daily dose of the drug in micrograms

$$150 \text{ microgram} \times 25 = 3750 \text{ micrograms}$$

Convert the total daily dose into mg

$$\frac{3750 \text{ micrograms}}{1000} = 3.75 \, mg$$

4. Calculate how much fluid the patient will need in one day

$$30 \, ml \times 65 = 1950 \, ml$$

Convert the volume into L

$$\frac{1950 \, ml}{1000} = 1.95 \, L$$

5. Calculate how much the patient will take in one day.

$$20 \, ml \times 4 = 80 \, ml$$

Calculate how much the patient will need for 30 days

$$80 \, ml \times 30 = 2400 \, ml$$

Convert the volume into L

$$\frac{2400 \, ml}{1000} = 2.4 \, L$$

6. **Step 1**: Work out what the ratio strength means

$$\text{Potassium permanganate 1 in 10,000} = 1 \, g \text{ in } 10,000 \, ml$$

Step 2: Convert the strength of solution to mgs

$$1 \, g \text{ in } 10,000 \, ml = 1 \times 1000 \, mg \text{ in } 10,000 \, ml$$

$$= 1000 \, mg \text{ in } 10,000 \, ml$$

Step 3: Calculate how much potassium permanganate there is in 100 ml of the solution

$$\frac{100}{10000} \times 1000 = 10 \, mg$$

7. **Step 1**: Work out what the percentage strength means in gram per 100 ml

Hydrogen peroxide 6% solution contains 6 g hydrogen peroxide in 100 ml solution

Step 2: Calculate how much hydrogen peroxide there is in 250 ml of the solution

$$\frac{250}{100} \times 6 = 15 \text{ g in } 250 \text{ ml}$$

8. You have levomepromazine injection 25 mg in 1 ml.

   Step 1: Calculate the volume of solution that contains 6.25 mg levomepromazine.

   $$\frac{6.25}{25} \times 1 \text{ ml} = 0.25 \text{ ml}$$

9. **Step 1**: Calculate the total dose of the drug.

   $$25 \text{ mg} \times 18 = 450 \text{ mg}$$

   Step 2: Calculate the volume of mixture that contains 450 mg.

   Mixture contains 200 mg in 5 ml

   Therefore, the volume that contains 450 mg will be:

   $$\frac{450}{200} \times 5 \text{ ml} = 11.25 \text{ ml}$$

10. You want to give a bolus dose of 100 mg lidocaine to a patient to control ventricular arrhythmia. The injection solution you have is lidocaine injection 2%. What volume of the injection do you need to give this dose?

    Step 1: Work out what the percentage strength means in gram per 100 ml

    Lidocaine 2% injection contains 2 g lidocaine in 100 ml solution.

    Step 2: Convert the strength of solution to mg in 100 ml

    $$2 \text{ g in } 100 \text{ ml} = 2 \times 1000 \text{ mg in } 100 \text{ ml}$$
    $$= 2000 \text{ mg in } 100 \text{ ml}$$

    Step 3: Calculate the volume of lidocaine injection that will contain 100 mg

    $$\frac{100}{2000} \times 100 \text{ ml} = 5 \text{ ml}$$

11. a. What is the IBW for a male who is 185 cm tall?

    Male: IBW $= (0.9 \times \text{height in cm}) - 88 \text{ kg}$
    $$= (0.9 \times 185) - 88 \text{ kg}$$
    $$= (166.5) - 88 \text{ kg}$$
    $$= 78.5 \text{ kg}$$

    Note: remember to multiply the numbers in brackets before you subtract the 88 kg

11. b. What is the IBW for a female who is 150 cm tall?

Female: IBW $= (0.9 \times$ height in cm$) - 92$ kg

$$= (0.9 \times 150) - 92 \text{ kg}$$

$$= (135) - 92 \text{ kg}$$

$$= 43 \text{ kg}$$

12. What is the dose of co-amoxiclav suspension 125/35 for a child aged 3 years weighing 16 kg? Use the dose stated in ml/kg body weight from your NPF or BNF (BNF, 2003).

BNF dose: 0.8 ml/kg daily given in three divided doses, increased to 1.6 ml/kg daily in three divided doses for severe infections. Choose 0.8 ml/kg daily.

Calculate the total daily dose:

Daily dose at 0.8 ml/kg $=$ Patient's weight (kg) $\times$ Daily dose (ml/kg)

$$= 16 \text{ kg} \times 0.8 \text{ ml/kg}$$

$$= 12.8 \text{ ml/day}$$

Calculate the dose to be given three times a day

$$= \frac{12.8 \text{ ml}}{3}$$

$$= 4.267 \text{ ml}$$

$$= 4.3 \text{ ml (rounded up to a practical dose)}$$

13. Calculate the dose of tobramycin for an adult female to treat a severe infection to be given by slow IV bolus injection. The dose recommended in the BNF (BNF, 2003) is 5 mg/kg daily in divided doses every 6 to 8 hours. The dose must be based on IBW. The patient is 165 cm tall.

Calculate the IBW:

Female: IBW $= (0.9 \times$ height in cm$) - 92$ kg

$$= (0.9 \times 165) - 92 \text{ kg}$$

$$= (148.5) - 92 \text{ kg}$$

$$= 56.5 \text{ kg}$$

Calculate the total daily dose:

Total daily dose at 5 mg/kg $=$ Patient's IBW (kg) $\times$ daily dose (mg/kg)

$$= 56.5 \text{ kg} \times 5 \text{ mg/kg}$$

$$= 282.5 \text{ mg}$$

Either calculate the dose to be given every 8 h:

$$= \frac{282.5}{3}$$

$$= 94.17 \text{ mg (rounded to 95 mg)}$$

Or calculate the dose to be given every 6 h:

$$= \frac{282.5}{4}$$

$$= 70.63 \, mg \text{ (rounded to 70 mg)}$$

Convert to a practical dose for administration to the patient:

If tobramycin injection contains 40 mg in 1 ml, the two doses above would equate to:

$$\textbf{Either } 95 \, mg \text{ every 8 h} = \frac{95}{40} \times 1ml = 2.375 \, ml$$

$$\textbf{Or } 70 \, mg \text{ every 6 h} = \frac{70}{40} \times 1ml = 1.75 \, ml$$

14. Calculate the dose of cyclophosphamide using the low-dose IV regimen for an adult patient with a BSA estimated at 1.95 m². The selected dose is 120 mg/m² once a week.

Weekly dose of cyclophosphamide $= 120 \, mg/m^2 \times 1.95 \, m^2$

$$= 234 \, mg$$

15. A patient requires 1 L of normal saline to be given over 12 hours. What is the correct rate for the drip controller in drops per minute assuming the giving set delivers 20 drops for 1 ml of solution?

$$1 L \text{ saline over } 12 \, h = \frac{1000 \, ml}{12} = 83.3 \, ml/h$$

$$83.3 \, ml/h = \frac{83.3}{60} = 1.39 \, ml/min$$

This could be rounded up to 1.4 ml/min.

20 drops = 1 ml, therefore 1.4 ml = 1.4 × 20 = 28 drops/min.

Therefore the drip rate controller should be set so that it administers 28 drops in one minute.

16. A patient requires 500 ml glucose 5% to be given over 3 hours. What is the correct rate for the drip controller in drops per minute assuming the giving set delivers 20 drops for 1 ml of solution?

$$500 \, ml \text{ glucose } 5\% \text{ over } 3 \, h = \frac{500}{3} = 166.7 \, ml/h$$

$$166.7 \, ml/h = \frac{166.7}{60} = 2.8 \, ml/min$$

20 drops = 1 ml, therefore 2.8 ml = 2.8 × 20 = 56 drops/min

Therefore the drip rate controller should be set so that it administers 56 drops in one minute.

17. Calculate the rate of administration in ml per hour of dobutamine infusion to be administered at a rate of 2.5 micrograms/kg/min to a patient weighing 75 kg. The solution should be made up (according to the IV monograph for critical care areas) as Dobutamine 250 mg in 500 ml NaCl 0.9% infusion.

2.5 micrograms/kg/min for a 75 kg patient = 2.5 × 75 micrograms/min
= 187.5 micrograms/min

187.5 micrograms/min = 187.5 × 60 micrograms/h = 11,250 micrograms/h

Convert to mg/h: 1000 micrograms = 1 mg

Therefore: 11,250 micrograms/h = 11.25 mg/h

Solution contains 250 mg dobutamine in 500 ml saline, how much does it contain in 1 ml?

$$250\,mg\ in\ 500\,ml = \frac{1\,ml}{500\,ml} \times 250\,mg = 0.5\,mg\ in\ 1\,ml$$

What volume will contain 11.25 mg?

$$\frac{11.25\,mg}{0.5\,mg} \times 1\,ml = 22.5\,ml/h$$

Therefore the pump should be set to administer 22.5 ml/h

18. Calculate the rate of administration in ml per hour of dopamine infusion to be administered at a rate of 2 micrograms/kg/min to a patient weighing 65 kg. The solution should be made up (according to the IV monograph) as Dopamine 800 mg in 500 ml fluid.

2 micrograms/kg/min in a patient weighing 65 kg = 130 micrograms/min

130 micrograms/min × 60 = 7800 micrograms/h

Convert to mg/h: 1000 micrograms = 1 mg

Therefore: 7800 micrograms = 7.8 mg

Dopamine solution contains 800 mg in 500 ml, how much does it contain in 1 ml?

$$\frac{1\,ml}{500\,ml} \times 800\,mg = 1.6\,mg\ in\ 1\,ml$$

$$\frac{7.8\,mg}{1.6\,mg} \times 1\,ml = 4.875\,ml/hr$$

Therefore the pump should be set to administer 4.88 ml/h

19. Calculate the dose of aminophylline infusion to treat an adult with an acute severe asthma attack. Assume that the patient has not previously been treated with theophylline or aminophylline. The patient weighs 65 kg. You need to prescribe a loading dose of 5 mg/kg given over 20 min then a maintenance dose of 500 micrograms/kg/h. The solution of aminophylline is made up as 500 mg in 500 ml.

Loading Dose

5 mg per kg × 65 kg = 325 mg over 20 min in either normal saline or glucose 5% infusion.

Maintenance Dose

500 micrograms/kg/h in a patient weighing 65 kg = 500 × 65 micrograms/h

$$= 32{,}500 \text{ micrograms/h}$$

$$\text{Convert to mg/h} = 32.5 \text{ mg/h}$$

The solution contains 500 mg in 500 ml, or 1 mg in 1 ml

Therefore the maintenance infusion should be set at 32.5 ml/h.

20. What is the cost per tablet of each of these drugs (rounded to nearest whole number)?

Ibuprofen 400 mg   £2.46 = 246/84 = 3 pence

Diclofenac 50 mg   £3.67 = 367/84 = 4 pence

Naproxen 500 mg   £3.08 = 308/28 = 11 pence

What is the cost per treatment day of each of these drugs (rounded to nearest whole number)?

Ibuprofen 400 mg   3 pence × 3 a day = 9 pence

Diclofenac 50 mg   4 pence × 3 a day = 12 pence

Naproxen 500 mg   11 pence × 2 a day = 22 pence

What is the cost per treatment course of each of these drugs?

Ibuprofen 400 mg   9p pence × 28 days = 252 pence = £2.52

Diclofenac 50 mg   12 pence × 28 days = 336 pence = £3.36

Naproxen 500 mg   22 pence × 28 days = 616 pence = £6.16

21. What is the cost per treatment day of each of these antacids (rounded to one decimal place)?

Cost/ml of liquid:

Algicon   £3.07 = 307 p/500 = 0.6 p/ml

Gastrocote   £2.67 = 267 p/500 = 0.5 p/ml

Gaviscon   £2.70 = 270 p/500 = 0.5 p/ml

Gaviscon Advance   £6.44 = 644 p/500 = 1.3 p/ml

Dosage per day:

Algicon   (20 × 4) = 80 ml

Gastrocote   (15 × 4) = 60 ml

Gaviscon   (20 × 4) = 80 ml

Gaviscon Advance   (10 × 4) = 40 ml

Cost per day of liquid:

Algicon	0.6 p per ml × 80 ml = 48 p
Gastrocote	0.5 p per ml × 60 ml = 30 p
Gaviscon	0.5 p per ml × 80 ml = 40 p
Gaviscon Advance	1.28 p per ml × 40 ml = 51 p

What is the cost per treatment course of each of these antacids?

Algicon	48 p × 28 days = £13.44
Gastrocote	30 p × 28 days = £8.40
Gaviscon	40 p × 28 days = £11.20
Gaviscon Advance	51 p × 28 days = £14.28

22.

Drug	Half-life (h)	Time to steady state plasma concentration (4–5 times half-life) (h)
Paracetamol	2	8–10
Indomethacin	2.4	9.6–12
Meloxicam	20	80–100
Piroxicam	48	192–240

23. After one half-life (8 h), theophylline level will have reduced by half.

$$\frac{28\ mg/L}{2} = 14\ mg/L$$

This lies within the reference range of 10–15 mg/L

24. **Step 1**: Phenytoin sodium capsule 100 mg = phenytoin liquid 90 mg

Step 2: Phenytoin sodium capsule (3 × 100 mg) + (1 × 50 mg)

$\qquad$ = phenytoin liquid (3 × 90 mg) + (1 × 45 mg)

$\qquad$ = phenytoin liquid 315 mg

Step 3: Phenytoin liquid contains 30 mg phenytoin in 5 ml. Therefore what volume contains 315 mg?

$$\frac{315\ mg}{30\ mg} \times 5\ ml = 52.5\ ml$$

25. **Step 1**: Total daily dose of carbamazepine = 400 mg × 2 = 800 mg

Step 2: Convert 800 mg orally to the equivalent in suppositories

$\qquad$ 100 mg orally = 125 mg rectally

Therefore, 800 mg orally = (8 × 125 mg) rectally

$$= 1000\,\text{mg}$$

Step 3: No more than 250 mg can be given at a time by the rectal route. Therefore a rectal dose of 1000 mg must be given as 250 mg four times a day.

26. **Step 1**: Calculate the amount of each ingredient:

Diamorphine = 50 mg in 2 ml water for injections (as stated)

Metoclopramide injection contains 10 mg in 2 ml

Therefore, metoclopramide 40 mg = 8 ml

Levomepromazine injection contains 25 mg in 1 ml

Therefore, levomepromazine 12.5 mg = 0.5 ml

Step 2: Calculate the volume of water for injection required

Total volume of the final solution is stated as 17 ml.

Therefore the amount of water for injection will be:

$$17\,\text{ml} - 8\,\text{ml} - 0.5\,\text{ml} = 8.5\,\text{ml}$$

Therefore the patient would need a supply of 10 ml ampoules of water for injection which do appear in the Drug Tariff and have now been added to the independent nurse prescribers' formulary.

27. **Step 1**: Calculate the total daily dose of morphine:

$$60\,\text{mg} \times 2 = 120\,\text{mg}$$

Step 2: Calculate the breakthrough dose of morphine

$$\frac{120\,\text{mg}}{6} = 20\,\text{mg}$$

A dose of 20 mg non-slow-release morphine should be prescribed, usually taken every four hours or more often according to patient need.

29. **Step 1**: Calculate the total daily dose of non-slow-release morphine

15 mg every 4 h = 15 mg × 6 = 90 mg

Step 2: Calculate the equivalent dose of slow-release morphine:

$$\frac{90\,\text{mg}}{2} = 45\,\text{mg twice a day}$$

Step 1: 90 mg morphine = 25 micrograms fentanyl/h

Step 2: Total daily dose of morphine = (120 × 2) mg = 240 mg

Step 3: Equivalent dose of fentanyl patch:

$$240\,\text{mg/day oral morphine} = \frac{240}{90} \times 25 = 66.6\,\text{micrograms}$$

Step 4: Find the nearest whole patch

A 75 micrograms/h patch would provide 8.4 micrograms more than calculated.

A 50 micrograms/h patch would provide 16.6 micrograms less than calculated.

30. **Step 1**: Total daily morphine $= (90\,\text{mg} \times 2) + (30\,\text{mg} \times 4) = 300\,\text{mg}$

Step 2: Sub-cutaneous does of diamorphine $= \dfrac{300\,\text{mg}}{3} = 100\,\text{mg}.$

Chapter 13

Prescribing in practice: how it works

Polly Buchanan

INTRODUCTION

Williams (1997) cites that at least 25% of the total population in the UK has a skin complaint of which 19% will consult their General Practitioner (GP). Therefore, caring for patients with dermatological conditions represents a significant workload for health professionals in primary care. Future dermatology services are aimed at improving dermatology services within primary care (Evans, 2001) and reducing the waiting times for patients to be seen in secondary care (Irvine, 2003). This has already resulted in the development of nurse-led clinics in primary care for patients with chronic inflammatory skin disease (Bowcock and Bailey, 2002; Mateos, 2002; Penzer, 2000; Rolfe, 2002a). Eczematous conditions, psoriasis and acne represent the three main chronic relapsing diseases, which can be managed more effectively in a primary care setting (Rolfe, 2002a).

Recent legislative changes surrounding the prescription of medications will enable nurse-led clinics and pharmacy services to complement GP and secondary care dermatology services (Bowman, 2000; DoH, 1999; 2000; 2002; 2003; Medicines Control Agency, 2002). For example, some of the topical and systemic medications used in dermatology are now available for nurses to prescribe independently. Furthermore, the advent of supplementary prescribing has meant that both nurses and pharmacists are able to prescribe from practically the whole of the British National Formulary (BNF) for patients with dermatological conditions through the use of Clinical Management Plans (CMPs).

The competency frameworks such as those developed by the National Prescribing Centre (NPC, 2001), the Nursing and Midwifery Council (NMC, 2003) and National Health Services (NHS) Scotland (NHS Education for Scotland, 2003) have enabled practitioners to acquire general prescribing competencies and those specific to dermatology in order for them to work competently in the role of prescriber. These include competencies in relation to:

- Clinical assessment of the patient's skin.

- Assessment of the patient's physiological, psychological and emotional response to a given dermatological diagnosis.

- Assessment of the patients response to therapeutic interventions and so the implementation of effective and safe therapeutic interventions.
- Provision of support and information regarding skin care.

This chapter describes how independent and supplementary prescribing can be used by non-medical prescribers in the treatment management of patients with dermatological conditions. It is hoped that readers will be provided with valuable insights with regard to how these modes of prescribing can be used to enhance patient care in other areas of practice and optimise the role of the non-medical practitioners involved in prescribing.

SKIN CARE

We are exposed to the concept of skin care on a daily basis. The cosmetic industry encourages everyone to care for his or her skin to aid attractiveness and prevent ageing. Many cosmetics and beauty products are designed specifically for skin. Fashion and beauty industries have made our expectations of having beautiful skin integral to our psyche. The 'look' of our skin affects our self-esteem. Therefore, it is important that healthcare professionals, involved in caring for patients with skin-related disease, as well as having a basic understanding of the anatomy and physiology of normal skin and knowledge of common dermatoses, also appreciate the effects of overt skin disease on self-image and how important it is to provide adequate care for these individuals (Papadopoulos and Bor, 1999).

PRESCRIBING FOR PATIENTS WITH DERMATOLOGICAL CONDITIONS

The skin is the largest vital organ of the body and can be effectively treated via the transcutaneous route. Therefore, the majority of medications used in dermatology are topical. Although many medicines still remain within the remit of the consultant dermatologist and the GP to prescribe, a number of preparations are available to independent extended nurse prescribers (Table 13.1). The advent of supplementary prescribing has also facilitated therapeutic interventions for a number of further dermatological conditions for non-medical prescribers. These include psoriasis (chronic plaque, guttate, scalp and flexural), rosacea, blistering conditions, drug eruptions, pruritus, pre-cancerous skin lesions (actinic keratoses), pityriasis and juvenile plantar dermatosis.

MAJOR FACTORS INFLUENCING THE USE OF TOPICAL AND SYSTEMIC MEDICATIONS IN DERMATOLOGY

The greatest benefits of topical medications are the safety profiles (low potential for systemic absorption/toxicity), efficacy profiles (good transcutaneous absorption), minimal side-effects and cost-effectiveness. However, the greatest disadvantages of topical medications used in dermatology relate to the odour, the appearance, the consistency, the frequency of application and staining of skin, hair, furniture and clothes. These disadvantages are incongruent with patient concordance.

Table 13.1　Skin conditions for which independent extended nurse prescribers are able to prescribe

Abrasions
Acne
Boil/carbuncle
Burn/scald
Candidiasis
Chronic skin ulcer
Dermatitis (atopic, contact, seborrhoeic)
Dermatophytosis of the skin (ringworm)
Herpes labialis
Impetigo
Insect bites/stings
Lacerations
Nappy rash
Pediculosis (head lice)
Pruritus in chickenpox
Scabies
Urticaria
Warts (including verrucas)

(Nurse Prescribers Formulary (NPF), 2003–2005).

For example, patients with psoriasis and self-caring for their skin at home, frequently report difficulties in using tar-based or anthralin-based preparations. Although these medications are effective if used with support and education, it takes a very dedicated and motivated patient to use these products in the moderate and long term due to the staining of skin, clothes and furniture. Consideration and discussion of other less 'messy' topical preparations for psoriasis, such as vitamin D analogues, corticosteroids and retinoids, as other treatment options will demand further patient education. Therefore, before the patient is able to choose or agree to the appropriate medication, they require an understanding of such factors as the side-effects and the possibility of tachyphylaxis with long-term usage.

If the prescriber is to achieve patient concordance and so clinical effectiveness for patients with dermatological conditions, they must have a good general understanding of basic pharmacology and its application to the treatment management of these patients. This includes an understanding of how individual medicines exert their effect, and how individual differences alter this effect. This will enable decisions to be made about the route of administration of a drug, the dose and frequency, contraindications and adverse effects.

Furthermore, cure is not an anticipated treatment outcome for chronic relapsing skin disease such as psoriasis or eczema. Dermatological patients frequently report that the most difficult aspect of their skin condition is learning to live with it (Buchanan, 2001; McGuckin, 2003). It is therefore essential that the practitioner feels confident to help the patient manage their skin during a lifetime, reducing the severity of relapses and extending the periods of remission. Educator, advisor, assessor and auditor are each essential components within the prescriber's remit when prescribing for patients with skin disease. This can only be achieved if the patients' concerns, lifestyle, age, abilities and individual coping strategies are understood by the practitioner.

Patients with chronic relapsing skin disease have generally developed a deep understanding of their condition (Titman, 2001), i.e. how it affects their life and which treatment regimens are effective for them. If practitioners are to identify and select the most appropriate medication for the patient, their assessment must be holistic, including the physical, psychological, emotional, social and spiritual aspects of the disease. In order for this to happen, the expert knowledge that the patient brings to the assessment consultation must be shared with the healthcare professional. This will enable the patient to become a partner in their care and so greatly influence how they use the medications prescribed.

Information and advice provided by the prescriber to the patient represent the most important factors that influence the use of topical medication (Gradwell, 2001). Inadequate information and support during a treatment programme often results in misunderstanding, disillusionment and poor concordance by the patient (Buchanan, 1998; Davis, 2002; Noren, 1995; Titman, 2001). The length of time for medications to take effect (often weeks) and the nature of topical formulations further compound the problem of poor concordance.

Supplementary prescribing, with its strong focus on concordance, provides an ideal framework within which to prescribe medicines for these patients. Supplementary prescribing requires the patient's consent for the prescribing partnership between the independent (IP) and supplementary prescriber (SP) to go ahead, i.e. the patient's goals and beliefs must be placed at the centre of prescribing decisions.

The treatment management of acne vulgaris (discussed below) is used to demonstrate how independent and supplementary prescribing can be used by non-medical prescribers to enhance patient care.

ACNE VULGARIS

Acne vulgaris is an inflammatory condition which affects the pilo-sebaceous units of the skin. The face, neck, shoulders, chest and back are often affected and it is extremely common during adolescence and early adulthood. Acne vulgaris is characterised by an increase in sebum production, presence of open and closed comedones, and increase in the *Propionibacterium acnes* (*P. acnes*) organism in the sweat gland duct, increase in free fatty acids and inflammation around the sebaceous gland (Buxton, 1993). During the disease coarse lesions may vary from comedones, papules, pustules, cysts and scars.

THE TREATMENT MANAGEMENT OF ACNE VULGARIS

Prescribing for acne depends on severity and psychological impact the condition has on the patient (National Institute for Clinical Excellence (NICE), 2000). Mild acne may have such a devastating effect on the patient's self-esteem that active medical intervention is appropriate. Moderate to severe acne requires prompt medical intervention to prevent scarring and to control exacerbations (Papadopoulos and Bor, 1999). Management strategies relate to the pathology of the disease and incorporates anti-comedonal, anti-inflammatory antibacterial agents, and anti-androgen preparations (Cunningham, 2000; Rolfe, 2002b).

Topical retinoids, topical antimicrobials, topical antibiotics and systemic antibiotics are preparations used to treat mild to moderate comedonal and inflammatory acne vulgaris (British Association of Dermatologists (BAD), 2004; Gollnick and Cunliffe, 2003). Nurses are able to prescribe for this condition independently or, as a SP, depending on their level of competence. Although General Sales List (GSL) and pharmacist only (P) medications can be recommended to the patient and supplied by the pharmacists, supplementary prescribing can also be used by pharmacists to prescribe for this condition.

As outlined above, CMPs are an essential component of supplementary prescribing. Figure 13.1 outlines a CMP that might be used for the management of mild to moderate acne.

TREATMENT COMPLICATIONS

Complications that may arise when treating patients with acne vulgaris surround poor patient concordance, i.e. intermittent application, antibiotic resistance, and irritancy. For example, managing the comedonal component of acne is fundamental in the treatment management of this condition. Comedones and micro-comedones are the precursor lesions to the inflammatory papules and pustules of acne. Therefore, anti-comedonal therapies are an essential component of the overall treatment. Topical retinoids are the recommended group of drugs for comedonal acne. They are indicated for active therapeutic regimens and maintenance therapy and can be used as a monotherapy for uncomplicated comedonal acne but most often combination therapy is indicated with antimicrobial agents or antibacterials. Support and advice are essential when prescribing topical retinoids due to the irritation these preparations can cause. The irritant potential of the medication needs to be explained to the patient with mention of mild scaling, dryness and erythema. Advice on how applications can be titrated to reduce side-effects must also be provided.

Antibacterial agents, which may be prescribed by IP or SPs, help control colonisation of *P. acnes* the organism responsible for mediating the inflammatory response in acne. Resistance of *P. acnes* is increasing, therefore, prescribing of antibiotics is restricted to cases which are unresponsive to antibacterial agents. Prescribing different topical and systemic antibiotics concurrently is not recommended (Nurse Prescribers Formulary (NPF), 2003). Prolonged or continuous courses of antibiotics encourage resistance. Therefore, courses should be adequate to treat the condition and then discontinued (Nurse Prescribers Formulary (NPF), 2003). Topical antibiotics should be continued for at least 6 months. Systemic antibiotics are

Name of patient: Miss Y	Patient medication sensitivities/allergies: None known

| Patient identification, e.g. ID number, date of birth: 21/2/85 | |

IP(s): DR G	SP(s) Sister A

Condition(s) to be treated	Aim of treatment
Acne vulgaris	To reduce, control and prevent comedonal, seborrhoeic and inflammatory components of acne with minimal side-effects. To reduce scarring.

Medicines that may be prescribing by SP:

Preparation Mild	Indication	Dose schedule	Specific indications for referral back to the IP
1 Topical retinoids	Reduction and control of comedonal lesions and inflammatory lesions in mild to moderate acne	As detailed in: BNF Section 13.6.1 topical preparations for acne	
+			
2 Topical antimicrobials	Reduction and control of comedonal and inflammatory lesions in mild to moderate acne	As above	Diagnosis in doubt
Moderate			
+/−3 Systemic antibiotics	Reduction and control of inflammatory acne of moderate severity	BNF sction 13.6.2 oral antibacterials for acne	Failure to respond to treatment
+/−4 Systematic anti-androgen	Reduction and control of seborrhoeic component in moderate acne	As above	

Guidelines or protocols supporting CMP:

Consult local formulary guidelines for first choice of topical and systemic drugs (practitioner would be required to reference these guidelines in the CMP)

BNF prescribing guidelines

BAD Guidelines (British Association of Dermatologists)

Frequency of review and monitoring by:

SP as indicated by response 1–3 monthly	SP and IP No less than 6 monthly

Process for reporting ADRs:

Yellow Card system. Verbal and written reporting by SP to IP

Shared record to be used by IP and SP:

Nurse led clinic documentation (integrated care pathway and clinical assessment records) as well as computerised patient records within surgery or practice

Agreed by IP(s)	Date	Agreed by SP(s)	Date	Date agreed with patient/carer

Figure 13.1   CMP for mild to moderate acne

reserved for cases where topical medications were ineffective. An oral course of antibiotics should demonstrate a response at3 months with maximum effect between 4 and 6 months. If there is no adequate response at 3 months another systemic antibiotic should be considered (Nurse Prescribers Formulary (NPF), 2003). It is vital that patients are provided with the appropriate information about their condition and the antibacterial therapy in order that patient concordance is increased and the risk of antibacterial resistance is reduced.

Whether prescribing independently or as a SP it is clear that the patient with acne vulgaris must be involved in the prescribing decisions that are made. As already highlighted, information and advice provided by the prescriber to the patient, represent the most important factors that influence the use of topical medication (Gradwell, 2001). As supplementary prescribing requires consent by the patient for the prescribing partnership to go ahead, this mode of prescribing with its strong focus on concordance, provides an excellent framework for the treatment management of this condition and should improve patient adherence to treatment regimes.

CONCLUSION

This chapter has discussed some of the key issues involved in the prescription of medicines for patients with skin disease and specifically acne vulgaris. Some of the major influencing factors in the use of topical and systemic medications for these conditions have been outlined. Although nurses are able to prescribe independently for a number of dermatological conditions, supplementary prescribing has enabled both nurses and pharmacists to prescribe for many additional skin diseases.

Information and advice represent the most important factors influencing the use of topical medication by patients with dermatological conditions (Acne Support Group, 2004). Supplementary prescribing, with its strong focus on concordance, provides an ideal framework within which to prescribe medicines for these patients.

References

Acne Support Group (2004). Patient information www.stopspots.org

Bowman J (2000). Nurse prescribing in a day-care dermatology unit. *Professional Nurse* **15(9)**: 573–577.

Bowcock S, Bailey K (2002). The introduction of nurse led clinics in dermatology. *British Journal of Dermatology Nursing* **1(4)**: 22.

British Association of Dermatologists (2004a). Acne Guidelines www.bad.org.uk/doctors/guidelines/acne.asp

British Association of Dermatologists (2004b). Acne Guidelines www.bad.org.uk/patients/disease/acne.asp

Buchanan PJ (2001). Behaviour modification: a nursing approach for young children with atopic eczema. *Dermatology Nursing* **13(1)**: 15–25.

Buchanan PJ (1998). Dermatology: RCN continuing education series. *Nursing Standard* **12(40)**: 48–55.

Buxton PK (1993). *ABC of Dermatology*. London: British Medical Journal Publishing Group, pp. 39–43.

Cunningham M (2000). Effective acne treatment. *British Journal Dermatology Nursing* **4(4)**: 12–15.

Davis R (2002). Caring for the skin at home. In: *Nursing Care of the Skin* (Penzer) Oxford: Butterworth-Heinemann. Chapter 5: pp. 116–142.

Department of Health (1999). *Review of Prescribing, Supply and Administration of Medicines. Final Report (The Crown Report)*. London: DoH.

Department of Health (2000). *The NHS Plan: A Plan for Investment. A Plan for Reform*. London: The Stationery Office.

Department of Health (2002). *Extending Independent Nurse Prescribing within the NHS in England. A Guide for Implementation*. London: DoH.

Department of Health (2003). *Supplementary Prescribing by Nurses and Pharmacists within the NHS in England: A Guide for Implementation*. London: DoH.

Gollnick H, Cunliffe W *et al.* (2003). Management of acne: Report from a global alliance to improve outcome in acne. *Journal of the American Academy of Dermatology* (Supplement) **49(1)**: S1–S37.

Gradwell C (2001). How to … Meet the educational needs of a dermatology patient. *British Journal of Dermatology Nursing* **5(4)**: 12–13.

Mateos M (2002). The health visitor role in setting up a nurse-led eczema clinic. *Dermatological Nursing* **1(4)**: 6–8.

McGuckin F (2003). My journey with psoriasis. *British Journal of Dermatology Nursing* **7(3)**: 14–15.

Medicines Control Agency (2002). *Proposals for Supplementary Prescribing by Nurses and Pharmacists and Proposed Amendments to the Prescription Only Medicines (Human Use) Order 1997*. London: DoH.

NHS Education for Scotland (2003). *Caring for People with Dermatology Conditions: A Core Curriculum. Quality Assuring Continuing Professional Education*. Edinburgh. www.qacpd.org.uk

National Institute of Clinical Excellence (2000). *GP Referral Practice: A Guide to Appropriate Referral from General to Specialist Services*. NHS NICE. www.nice.org.uk

National Prescribing Centre (2001). *Maintaining Competency in Prescribing. An Outline Framework to Help Nurse Prescribers*. Liverpool: NPC.

Nursing and Midwifery Council (2003). QA factsheet D6 www.nmc-uk.org/nmc/main/qa/docs/QA-c2003pdf

Noren P (1995). Habit reversal: a turning point in the treatment of atopic dermatitis. *Clinical and Experimental Dermatology* **20**: 2–5.

NPF (2003–2005). British Medical Association, Royal Pharmaceutical Society of Great Britain. In association with Community Practitioners' and Health Visitors' Association, Royal College of Nursing.

Papadopoulos L, Bor R (1999). *Psychological Approaches to Dermatology.* Leicester: The British Psychological Society. Chapter 1: pp. 1–6.

Papadopoulos L, Bor R (1999). *Psychological Approaches to Dermatology.* Leicester: The British Psychological Society. Chapter 11: pp. 122–123.

Penzer R (2000). Improving psoriasis care through a nurse-led service. *Community Nurse* **6(2)**: 12.

Rolfe G (2002a). A nurse-led acne, psoriasis and eczema initiative in Northants. *Dermatological Nursing* **1(4)**: 18–20.

Rolfe G (2002b). Nursing role for acne in primary care. *British Journal of Dermatology Nursing* **6(3)**: 9–11.

Titman P (2001). Understanding the stresses on mothers of children with eczema. *British Journal of Dermatology Nursing* **5(4)**: 7–9.

Williams H (1997). Dermatology. In: *Health Care Needs Assessment: The Epidemiologically Based Needs Assessment Reviews* 2nd edn (Stevens, A and Raftery, J) Oxford: Radcliffe Medical Press. Section 5: pp. 2–32.

Index